# finding zen
# with cancer

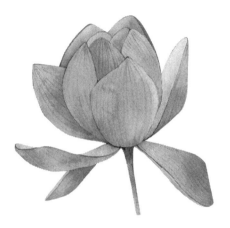

How My Stage 3 Cancer Diagnosis Healed My Life
and Led Me to My Soul's Calling

# Linda Christine Stansberry

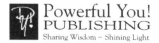

Powerful You!
PUBLISHING
Sharing Wisdom ~ Shining Light

# Finding Zen With Cancer

*How My Stage 3 Cancer Diagnosis Healed My Life and Led Me to My Soul's Calling*

Copyright © 2023

Published by: Powerful You! Inc. USA
powerfulyoupublishing.com

Library of Congress Control Number: 2023916921

Linda Christine Stansberry – First Edition
Dade City, Florida
findingzenwithcancer.blogspot.com

ISBN: 978-1-959348-18-4

First Edition October 2023

HEALTH & FITNESS / Diseases & Conditions / Cancer

# Dedication

This book is dedicated to all who supported me through my cancer journey, especially my loving life partner, Greg, and my dear children, Alex, Megan, Melissa, Hannah, and Noah.

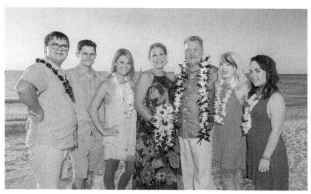

L to R: Noah, Alex, Hannah, Linda, Greg, Melissa, & Megan

Richard -
may your Zen always
be within reach!
all the best,
Linda

# Table of Contents

# Author's Note

There are many perspectives around healing. Consider for a moment (this one's gonna require you to dig down deep and move past all the triggers) that perhaps your cancer diagnosis was a gift.

It's easy for me to look back now and see how my diagnosis was the catalyst for my soul-shifting transformation to a state of higher consciousness. If you'd told me that during treatment, I would have likely been very triggered and definitely pissed off that you even went there. Now, however, after ten years on the other side of cancer, I can clearly see how this was a literal my *do-or-die moment.*

This book in no way offers medical advice. This memoir is merely my uncensored depiction of my cancer journey and my retrospective view on how my mind, body, and soul have evolved in the decade since.

I believe traumas and tragedies are great teachers, designed to show us the inner power and strength we never knew that we had. We have come here to be warriors, examples for those around us, pillars of strength that show those witnessing our journey that we are as strong (or as weak) as we believe we are.

I feel that we can all find lessons in the traumas we suffer, and it certainly becomes much easier once you're on the other side of that trauma.

As you venture down your own path of healing, you have two options:

1. Be the victim of a disease that was put upon you.

Or

2. Be the warrior-teacher-sage as you power through the pain toward your purpose.

I love you!
Linda

# Preface

I spent my formative years in my dream job, writing and producing commercials and promos for local TV stations in various cities around the country. I loved the creative process; it fed my soul.

After just over a decade as a creative, I felt obligated to take the next step into management. The lure of a bigger salary and the idea that managing creatives would be fun was all I needed to solidify that decision. If only it was that simple.

My first upper-management gig was a deep dive into the ugly truths of corporate mandates: first and foremost, please the shareholders at all costs. Those "costs" were at the expense of the workers in the form of hiring freezes, zero pay increases, and skyrocketing out-of-pocket health care costs each year. Meanwhile, the TV cash cow kept serving up rich milk to the shareholders, who loved scraping the creamy sixty percent profit margins off the top.

Fast forward twenty years. I was trudging through my second Creative Director position and was even less enamored with the corporate lifestyle of upper management. I spent more time managing up than down, I was exposed to all the seedy dealings that were sold to me as legit, I was judged because I was not heavy-handed with my staff (a horrible way to deal with creative types), and I was stabbed in the back daily by staff as well as by my boss and other department heads.

This quote from Hunter S. Thompson's *Generation of Swine: Tales of Shame and Degradation in the '80s* was a favorite among us in the television business:

> The TV business is uglier than most things. It is normally perceived as some kind of cruel and shallow money trench through the heart of the journalism industry, a long plastic hallway where thieves and pimps run free and good men die like dogs, for no good reason.

As if this wasn't enough, my second marriage to my first husband was eroding quickly. Yes, you read that correctly: my *second* marriage to my *first* husband. Some lessons are hard-learned for this gal.

My husband was struggling with anger issues along with his unmanaged sobriety, which created a "dry drunk" scenario in our house. Essentially, we were struggling with all the behaviors of an alcoholic husband/father, minus the alcohol. He was quite willing to address the aforementioned issues once I asked for a divorce. For me, it was too little, too late.

The marriage finally ended for good one evening when he was taken to jail on a domestic assault charge, which resulted in felony charges because he took my phone away from me as I called 911. All this in front of our nine-year-old Asperger's child.

He threatened to call my work and degrade me to my co-workers and management. I had to have his photo posted at the front desk in case he showed up. So, basically, he won. I *was* feeling quite degraded at this point.

I spent the next eighteen months trying to finalize the divorce. I was feeling depressed, defeated, and DONE. Done with all the drama that I had to manage daily in my work life as well as my home life. Done with believing that my life could ever be filled with peace. Done with the idea that there was a partner out there for me that didn't require me to coddle, conform to, or align with their trauma.

Then one day my life took an upturn. I was scrolling social media and saw Greg, my high school sweetheart, pop up on a post.

Mind you, this wasn't a passing fling but an intense on-and-off-again romance that stretched from our teens into our early twenties. He eventually joined the Navy as I was transitioning into my second TV job. The stars didn't align for us to take our relationship to the next step. We were both maneuvering the challenges of trying to find our place in the world. But he remained in my heart. Always.

After I found him online, Greg and I began writing each other. He was struggling with a soon-to-be-empty nest and looking headlong at a marriage that held no future for him. The only thing he felt he and his wife had in common was their two daughters.

He was able to amicably finalize his divorce within two months. Meanwhile, mine was still dragging on; however, I felt my life was certainly looking up with Greg in the picture.

I finally had life by the balls...that is, until the dreaded "c" word entered, stage three.

This memoir is my look back on my cancer journey then and now, a decade after the diagnosis. It is a no-holds-barred, raw, and raucous account of my search for my zen within this diagnosis. I journaled my way through treatment, then, and now, offering prayers and meditations each step of the way.

My intention for this book is to inspire, illuminate, and expand the minds of those embarking on their own cancer journey, as well as offer perspective for loved ones and caregivers of cancer patients.

It is important to note: this book does NOT contain any medical advice. This is purely my journey, in my own words. So, if you're willing to embrace an honest depiction of the ugly truths and the deep dives, along with the lighter side of cancer treatment and the heart-centered, spiritual revelations uncovered throughout the journey, then this book is for you!

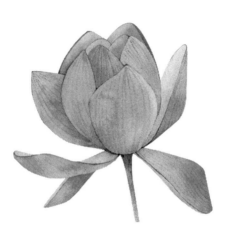

# Chapter One
# My Pre-Cancer Vision

**Blog Post: March 18, 2013**

My life is definitely on the upswing.

- I left an abusive marriage, now I am finally beginning to dig my way out of two years of financial rubble (thanks to the weight of exorbitant alimony payments).
- I am creating a peaceful home for my children.
- I am being challenged at work and, given the circumstances, feel I am successfully rising to the occasion.
- I am a health club member and have been since 2012.
- I am happy that I am getting some long overdue rehab after my 2011 knee surgery, plus feeling good both physically *and* mentally.
- The best part of my life: I am reunited with my high school sweetheart after 24 years apart! I am finally having the relationship of my dreams.

The very next day, March 19th, that vision would be abruptly ripped away. Suddenly, I was living in a tenuous world. I would soon become an outsider in my own body. My "normal" would disappear. My vision would morph into a weak and fragile depiction of a life I never imagined would be mine.

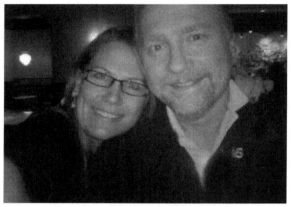

*Greg and me, December 2011*

It is interesting how hindsight can make one's life crystal clear. As I exited my marriage and entered into my relationship with Greg, I saw so much potential that I never knew (or believed) could exist for me. More accurately, the dream I'd held of finding that perfect-for-me mate had become foggy, like a distant memory.

A few years earlier, I'd gone on a cruise to Cozumel with my friend Karen (aka "Krisco"). One of the excursions we took was a day trip to Tulum to visit the Mayan Ruins.

Since the ruins were known as a sacred place for

Mayan ceremonies, I suggested that we both create a list of what we wanted in a partner and have our own ceremony. Then, while on the excursion, we would bury that list in one of the temples, asking the Mayan Gods to fulfill that list and deliver us our desired mate. So, of course, we did just that!

Later that same year, we each ended up in a relationship with a man who matched our list. Both of us are still with those men to this day.

At that time, my awareness was not as open and focused as it is today. However, I have always been a believer that there is a higher power (God/Source/ Creator) that watches after us. I have always believed in angels and felt a deep connection to the angelic realm. And I am certain that there is some guiding force that, if we are able to tune into that force, we can be guided on a serendipitous journey that leads us directly to our heart's desire, just like Penny Peirce's book, The Intuitive Way.

I was giddy like a schoolgirl, feeling so wonderfully blessed to have this reunion with the man that I loved decades ago. Yet, just beneath the surface of my giddiness was a thick layer of deep regret. Regret that we never followed through with our relationship years ago. Regret that we never had the opportunity to create a family together. Regret over what "could have been" is a deep, dark crevasse that can suck you quicker than a Florida sinkhole. I fell hard into that crevasse.

## *Prayer to Release Regret*

*God, wash over my human body and heavenly soul with release.*

*Release the deepest regrets that no longer serve who I am today.*

*I release any and all discordant energy to you, Oh Lord, to transmute into the highest form of love.*

*Dear Creator, illuminate me with your unconditionally loving light so that I may go forward with the resonance of harmony within my being and absolute peace in my soul.*

## Chapter Two
# Colonoscopy Numero Uno

**Blog post: March 19, 2013**

Today is my first colonoscopy. It is routine in the sense that I just turned forty-nine only thirteen days ago, and I am quickly approaching the mid-century mark. However, it's not so routine because colon cancer runs rampant in my family. My father and my mother's brother both died of colon cancer. Because of this, my primary care doc is adamant that I get a colonoscopy ASAP. He feels I am already long overdue. So here I am.

I go into this procedure with an open mind. Everyone will tell you the prep is the worst part, but for me, it is refreshing to feel 'light' around my midsection. Without being overly descriptive, either I'm "slow to move," or everything shoots through me all at once. Okay, okay, TMI, I know!

After the procedure, I am told that the colon doc removed five small to medium size polyps. Everyone appears a little surprised by the number of polyps, but they all assure me the polyps don't look abnormal to the naked eye.

This is the part where an annoying little voice in my head says, "Something's not right." I hate that voice. I work hard to dismiss any thoughts that are remotely negative. My life is going great! I kick that little voice to the curb and keep living my life. Status quo, baby!

I have always wondered if that little voice was my inner knowing, bracing me for the worst.

In general, the narrative that ran through my head twenty-four/seven was a non-stop stream of horrible, awful, no-good thoughts about every possible disaster that would likely happen to me, by me, or because of me. I honestly don't know how I lived my life in that state. Again, this is another nod to hindsight for providing amazing clarity.

My father passed from colon cancer on June 3, 1992. The very next day, I found out I was pregnant with my daughter, Hannah.

My parents split up when I was nine and ended up living on opposite ends of the Mississippi (my mom and I in Minnesota, my dad in New Orleans), yet Dad and I had remained very close.

Though he was far from perfect, he was perfect for me. He was always my biggest fan, my cheerleader. He never told me my dreams were impossible. And he supported my creativity; he even gifted me my first camera.

Dad always told me he wasn't prepared to have three kids in diapers when my mom was twenty-two years old. (My siblings—two sisters and a brother—had each arrived a year apart.) When I came along eleven years later (oops!), he said he was ready; or so his story goes.

When my parents split, I wasn't told about it. I simply packed my suitcase and went off to Minnesota with Mom, just as I did every year. Summer vacation turned into enrollment in school that fall. Then the holidays came and went. My intuition knew without a doubt that their marriage was over. Meanwhile, little Linda was left wondering why her dad was gone.

This was a heavy situation to lay on a nine-year-old, and even more so because it was so mismanaged. It had me inventing stories in my head. When my new circle of friends asked me where my dad was, I would say he went on frequent business trips. Lack of information certainly creates misinformation when it comes to a child's scared and worried mind. I don't blame my parents; I gave that up years ago. They did the best they could, given the lack of awareness they held at the time.

After our move, my dad and I never had much time together, so when we did, it truly seemed like quality time. Or perhaps it is just my conscious mind desperately grabbing hold of those times with such fervor that it would be impossible to forget.

Fast forward fifteen years, I remember vividly the

day my dad told me he "wouldn't be around much longer." He said it just like that.

He made the trip up to Minnesota that summer of 1989. We were sitting outside at Lord Fletcher's on Lake Minnetonka. He was drinking a glass of wine; I was likely having my standard rum and coke. Dad took my hand and placed it just under his left rib cage, and he placed it on a lump roughly the size of a large orange.

I freaked out. "Wait! What?! What is this?"

He calmly said, "I don't think your old man is going to be around much longer."

He went on to tell me he would be seeing a doctor soon. I was so upset with him for not having this checked sooner. The man literally ate antacids like they were candy, as hindsight showed me this problem had existed for quite a long time.

After his doctor's visit, he was told he needed surgery. Surgery consisted of opening him up, seeing all the cancer scattered throughout his insides, including his liver, and sewing him shut again.

Diagnosis: Stage 4 colon cancer, six months to live.

Reality: he lived another three years. The moral of this story: don't EVER let anyone put a date on your life. No one can predict your expiration date.

I still miss my dad terribly. I am so very grateful that he lived long enough to see his namesake, my son Alexander, born in 1990.

After my dad's passing, I saw how shallow and

unaware everyone seemed around me. The lack of empathy, and their ability to mercilessly move on. I now realize what I was seeing was not *in* everyone else. I was seeing my own reflection in a mirror, a virtual cosmic mirror that each and every one of those individuals held up for ME to look into and see my own shallowness and lack of awareness.

My father's death and my cancer year were the two most pivotal events in my life. Both of those situations profoundly shifted my consciousness. My soul literally up-leveled into a whole other realm of awareness.

### *Prayer of Reflection*

*Angels of Love and Light, show me the way to understanding as my humble existence is filled with frustration toward my fellow man.*

*Guide me to see all with your loving eyes,*

*Summon me so I may hear the sorrow of my own sadness in others,*

*Hold me so that I may know that the anger seemingly caused by others is truly my own pain reflected back to me.*

*This is a lesson for my earthly being to conquer.*

*This is a lesson for my earthly soul to embrace.*

*Thank you.*

## Chapter Three
# Hello, Bad News Here

**Blog Post: March 24, 2013**

Every other weekend my youngest goes to his dad's house. Alone time with my guy is a commodity, so we always make plans to do something special together. Saturday we plan to visit Travares, the seaplane capital of Florida, and Mt. Dora. On Sunday we head to Sarasota for brunch and shopping at the newly opened Trader Joe's.

Both days are fun-filled, spontaneous, and wonderful!

On Sunday, we ate an amazing meal at The Breakfast House. We purely stumbled upon this place by happenstance and it's now our favorite.

Next, we are off to the Shore Diner on Saint Armands Circle for our favorite, the bacon Bloody Mary!

I had just bellied up to the bar when my phone rings. It is my gastroenterologist. My heart stops. Why is a doctor calling a patient on Sunday? I quickly find out why. He asks if anyone called me to discuss my pathology report. I know immediately that this is bad news. My eyes well up with tears as he explains the results of the pathology report and how they want to treat this aggressively given my family history of colon cancer. He said the surgery I will need is rather routine and should get me cancer free in no time. Surgery?!? Damn.

I hang up the phone and can barely speak. Tears roll down my face. Everything around me becomes surreal. I look at Greg, his face has a look I have never seen before. I could barely form two simple sentences, "I have cancer. I need surgery." He leans over and holds me like a piece of fragile china. "I'm so scared," I whisper.

The rest of the day my mind races. How can I possibly tell my children I have cancer? How do I tell anyone I have cancer? I feel like people will never see me the same again. Will people somehow believe this was my fault? Is it my fault or just my real shitty genetics?

It is impossible to know what it feels like to be told you have cancer unless you've been told you have cancer.

Additionally, I would surmise that it is impossible to know how to tell people you have a cancer diagnosis until you've been put into the position of having to tell loved ones you have a cancer diagnosis. You just do what inherently feels right at the time.

As I sat with my diagnosis, I was dumbfounded. Cancer is a surreal experience. You run the spectrum of emotions from shock, fear, sadness, and disbelief, and, for some, it can end there. But if you're a fighter, you eventually pack up your pity party and move on to feelings of courage, the inner strength to fight, and a deep knowing you'll overcome cancer or at least die trying. However, for me, the latter comes a bit later in this story.

My thoughts then turned to Greg. The love of my life. We were so happy to be reunited. We learned so much about what we would and would not tolerate from our previous relationships that we felt ready to take on the world together, then this. My mind started reeling with how this would affect him, how this would affect us. Could he or would he be up for this challenge? Was I worth it? What a way to step into year three of our relationship.

I felt gross all over. I felt like my body had betrayed me. I felt my genetics were at fault. I couldn't see past blaming my body to what is so obvious to me now; this was the culmination of years (or even lifetimes) of unresolved regret and repressed anger. I know for some, this is a difficult idea to wrap your mind around or even triggering, but humor me for a minute.

Cancer definitely has emotional roots. Repressed anger, resentment, and regret love to manifest in the physical as cancer. These factors play into the disease just as much as stress hormones or a suppressed immune system do. If you don't believe me, take a moment to do a quick internet search on the subject. You may be amazed at the articles and papers written on this subject.

We can take this idea one step further: if you believe in reincarnation, it is highly likely that your soul has spent lifetimes gathering feelings of repressed anger, regrets, and resentments. If these emotions are reoccurring themes in your life now, and you have not consciously examined their origins, they may appear for you in the body as physical ailments or even cancer.

And if you really want to get deep, I would go so far as to say that your cancer is a "pain to purpose" scenario, meaning your physical pain unfolds a greater purpose for you in this lifetime. Perhaps it is as simple as your cancer journey becomes an example for another person, leading to their life-altering experience.

The leap from feeling betrayed by your body to cancer being a part of your soul's journey is a big one. You can't make this leap immediately, but over time, you may see this possibility unfold.

### Temple of Light Meditation

Sit in silence.

Focus on slow breaths.

Breath in for 4 counts, out for five.

Repeat the following out loud or to yourself in silence.

*"Dear human vessel,*

*I ask you for forgiveness.*
*I have misused you in the past.*
*You are a glorious gift from the Creator of All that Is.*
*And I celebrate you. "*

Now imagine beautiful, iridescent, golden-white light pouring down directly from God, in through the crown of your head, and filling up every organ, blood vessel, and cell of your body, from the top of your head to the bottoms of your feet. Feel the warmth of this golden-white Source Light. Feel how it is infused with such deeply profound unconditional love.

Just feel....

Sit quietly for several minutes and note all the feelings moving through your body in this now moment. Not the feelings in your head, feelings in your <u>body</u>. These feelings can be anything, so do not judge.

Just feel.

Now, as you come back from the feelings, breathe slowly back into your body. Feel your feet connected to the ground, feel a beautiful golden cord connecting you to the core of Mother Earth. Slowly open your eyes and come back from your meditation.

*\*This is a wonderful journal opportunity to write down what your body felt during this meditation. Do not judge; just write all that you're feeling from your heart.*

## Chapter Four
# Keep Calm
# and Fuck Cancer

**Blog Post: March 28, 2013**

Today is my consultation with the surgeon. My gastroenterologist recommended this guy since he did his wife's colon resection surgery. It seems everyone I run into at the med center has rave reviews on how he did their wife's, husband's, sister's, or grandpa's

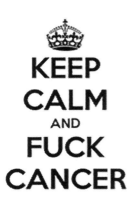 surgery and how he is so talented and wonderful. Using this guy sounds like a no-brainer.

Greg and my daughter attend my consult. I figure the more people I have listening to what the surgeon says, the better. We'll call him "Dr. N."

Dr. N. reviews my report and says I'll need to get another colonoscopy to "tattoo" the spot where the cancerous polyp was removed. As long as that spot is found and marked, Dr. N. will only need to remove nine inches of colon on either side; if not, he will remove a much larger section of my intestine. I feel fortunate when I find out Dr. N. is a skilled laparoscopic surgeon; otherwise, I'd have an equally long incision from my pubic bone up to the ribcage. Dr. N. went on to explain that they would test that section of the colon for cancer and make sure the cancer didn't work its way through the intestinal walls. Based on the report he was reading, he feels confident that wouldn't be the case.

I left the consultation thinking, *I can do this*. I can get this surgery complete and be done with the "C word." I also left  Dr. N's office forgetting to ask for the results of my CT Scan. I panicked for a moment, then realized I have multiple doctor's appointments over the course of the next few days. If it's important, surely someone will fill me in at some point.

The little voice popped up again and said, "It won't be good news."

"Fuck off, little voice," I replied.

❁ ❁ ❁ ❁ ❁

### Blog Post: March 30, 2013

It's a Saturday evening, the day before Easter. I'm at home, watching TV and relaxing after gorging myself at the Chinese buffet. Greg and I decided we'd do three days of buffets before I start my pre-colonoscopy and pre-surgery fasting on Monday.

My phone rings. I look at the number, and my stomach sinks into my knees…again. It's my workaholic, over-achieving colon doc calling me. God bless his work ethic, but come on, dude, spend some time with the wife and kids! It's Easter weekend, for Christ's sake! Of course, he is calling to say he was reviewing my CT scan results.

*Ugh, what now?* I thought.

He said my liver and kidney each had a little spot on them, which was completely normal and expected.

I'm waiting for the "but"…

He didn't see anything else in my intestines and they looked good.

I know the "but" is coming, just give it to me …

He could see that I'd had my gallbladder removed.

Duh. Get to the "but" …

But…

I KNEW IT!!

"I see a mass around your right ovary that gives me some concern."

I suddenly went deaf. The world around me was completely silent.

Was it really possible that I was being dealt a double dose of cancer?

I snapped out of it as the doc said he was writing instructions to his office so I could get an ultrasound of my ovaries on Monday. He then went on to explain that if it was cancer, I couldn't have my ovaries removed at the same time as my colon surgery; that procedure needed  to be done by a surgeon that specializes in ovarian cancer.

Great.

The rest of the night, I sat there as if the wind had been kicked out of me. Unable to clear my brain of all the what-ifs, I'm finding it increasingly harder to remain positive.

❁ ❁ ❁ ❁ ❁

## Blog Post: April 1, 2013

Pity the fool who decides to pull one over on me this day. I'm in <u>no</u> mood. Wait. I *am* in "a mood," but not the one all about the fun-filled trickery of April Fool's. I'm in a "Don't fuck with me, I'm wound so tight I could explode" mood, the kind that sends men and children running for the hills at the mere sight of me.

I found out Friday that I need to meet with my primary care doc for a pre-surgery physical...*today*! At this point, I'm wondering if there is anyone out there who isn't getting a piece of me.

The truth be told, I don't mind my doc, and my day is pretty much shot anyway. He is a cool guy with a good sense of humor and easy on the eyes. While I'm there, he listens to my heart and checks my breathing, and then we basically talk for thirty minutes straight. He tells me stories of cancer patients he's had, much younger than me, who have endured horrible bouts with the C word. Some even passed away. He all but promises me the mass they see on my ovaries will turn out to be nothing. We chat away like two college buddies talking baseball stats over beer, except *our* conversation revolves around cancer. All the while, it never dawns on me I could be one of "those people" who end up in one of his stories someday. In fact, I'm feeling overly optimistic as long as I can tamp down that annoying little voice inside my head.

An hour later, I'm downstairs getting the ultrasound of my ovaries.

"Are they kicking?" I ask.

The technician chuckles.

"It's much more exciting to see a fetus bouncing around in there!" I say.

After she rubs the probe around on my lower belly for a while, she then hands me a "special tool." This one is designed to see my ovaries from the *INSIDE*. Oh my, I suddenly feel like I'm in an episode of *Sex and the City*.

"Thanks, Samantha," I say while inserting the probe so the tech can take a closer look.

Afterward, as I smoke a cigarette and bask in the afterglow, I realize it's time to head home and begin yet another colon prep. Bye-bye, three days of buffet food.

Tests, tests, and more tests. This is how many

precancer treatment patients spend their days. It's frustrating, to say the least.

For those going through this process, I highly recommend surrounding yourself with upbeat, positive people to assist you. They will be your eyes, ears, and, most importantly, your cheerleaders through all the doctor's appointments you'll need to endure.

Caregivers, this is an exhausting process for the patient. Keep notes on all the appointments and keep the conversation light, no talk about anything cancer-related. At this point, we have overthunk it ad nauseam.

During all of this testing, I alternated between floating outside my body and feeling like this reality doesn't really exist to sitting hard in the reality of negative possibilities that this could be bad, really bad.

Fear was attached to me like the backpack of a kindergartener headed off to school. Everywhere I went, fear loomed. When I was supposed to be sleeping, fear barged in, clanging loud cymbals to make sure I knew it was there.

Later I learned that fear was a shitty friend. All it did was keep me distracted from my heart, fear blocked me from listening to what my soul wanted me to know. Fear was a horrible bedfellow. So, we eventually broke up.

### *Prayer Against the Unknown*

*I ask for gentle Angelic guidance as I embark into the darkness of the unknown.*

*I reach for you, God, and Your loving hand—cradle my uneasiness and transcend my fear with your Almighty strength.*

*I do not walk alone; I am surrounded by the loving energy of God's Army of Angels.*

*My heart swells with joyful anticipation,*

*I fall back into the abyss, trusting that I will be caught.*

*I know any and all outcomes*

*are for my highest and best good,*

*Even the outcomes that I may not understand.*

*I trust that my soul knows, this is the correct path.*

## Chapter Five
# Tattoo You,
# Surgery Day

**Blog Post: April 2, 2013**

I've been here so often that I'm friends with all the nurses at the Surgery Center. In fact, I'm now the Mayor on Foursquare (a social media app that shows I've been here waaaaayyy too much in the past thirty days!)

My favorite nurse who works with my colon doc (I hate that I can't remember her name!) was surprised to see me back again. She can't get over the fact I have cancer. She said, "We all looked at that polyp and said, nah…looks fine. I can't believe it came back with cancer!"

I asked to talk to my colon doc before they put me under. I knew he would have the results of my ultrasound. He did and THANK GOD, it's all good! He said the right ovary has a real gnarly, knotted-up cyst growing around it. Sounds lovely! He was sure Dr. N. would take pictures of it during surgery tomorrow, so we can keep an eye on it going forward.

Whew! What a relief!! One down, two to go!

When I awaken from my anal probing tattoo session, I am told the doctor easily found and marked the area where the cancerous polyp was removed two weeks ago. Another whew! He also found three more tiny polyps and diverticulitis. Seems to me that area of my colon is a hotbed for unwanted growths. I am starting to feel better about having that section removed.

❦ ❦ ❦ ❦ ❦

## Blog Post: April 3, 2013

Today is my descending colectomy laparoscopic surgery with urethral stints. In layman's terms, it's colon resection surgery. Now, let me answer the obvious question first. Yes, I am scared.

I've had six surgeries in my lifetime. They all took place just before and after the age of forty. My advice to everyone is don't turn forty because that's when the surgeries seem to start. For me, it began with a simple tubal ligation about a year after my youngest was born. My ex was chickenshit, so he never got around to getting a vasectomy—hence my third was born. I love all my kids deeply, but I did not want a fourth, and the tubal became necessary. That was followed by a bunionectomy on each foot, one in 2002 and one in 2003. After that, a partial hysterectomy in 2004 (I kept my ovaries since I wasn't ready for full-on menopause). Then, my gallbladder was removed around 2006, followed by my knee surgery in 2011.

All were done laparoscopically, for which I am very grateful!

Even after all those surgeries, I am still feeling quite apprehensive about this one. Hell, you'd think I would be a seasoned pro by now! It's the damn C word. For some reason, the word cancer changes EVERYTHING. In my mind, "The Force is with me." I believe I'll come out on the other side of this with a story to tell my grandkids someday. How could I not? The love of my

life is by my side, cheering me on every step of the way!

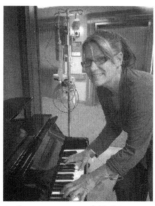

*Trying to keep my mood light post-surgery*

I wake up a few hours later. For the next twenty-four hours, I am floating in a morphine cloud. My Greg is sweet to update my social media page so everyone who is praying for me knows that I am OK. So far... so good! I do remember going in, but coming out, not so much. I'm still foggy...so foggy I was sure Greg said Dr. N. also took my ovaries out. Took my ovaries out, too? What? I know they aren't the most attractive ovaries based on my CT Scan, but take them out? Guess it's goodbye, cancer. Hello, menopause.

Post-surgery was rough—so much so it made the several previous procedures easy-breezy by comparison.

I still remember Greg telling me the doctor took my ovaries. I wasn't expecting it; I was sure we never discussed it at my consultation prior to surgery. At first, I was very upset; I was feeling betrayed, stripped of one of my last bits of womanhood. All chances of conceiving another child (even with a surrogate) were taken from me. I had always dreamed of what it would be like to have a child with Greg, a crazy dream for a forty-nine-year-old woman, I know, but … what if …?

After I came out of my post-surgical fog, I realized it was for the best. I was ready to be done with all this cancer BS, and if taking my ovaries lessened my chances of cancer coming back, then I was all for it.

Then there was the matter of the pain. Fortunately, my surgery was done laparoscopically, so I didn't have to deal with the pain of a large incision on top of it. But let me tell you, my belly button is a hot mess after all my laparoscopic surgeries!

If I can offer advice to anyone going through a

medical procedure, it's DO YOUR RESEARCH! I can't stress that enough. I believe I saved myself a WORLD of immeasurable pain by being on top of my post-surgery protocol. My nurse wanted to offer me a soda about four hours after having eighteen inches of my large intestine removed. I had read that you shouldn't have anything for at least the first twelve hours after surgery, or it could create serious pain. The nurse and I had a bit of a heated discussion over this— she eventually left and came back, deciding I *could* have ice chips. Needless to say, the rest of the night didn't go so well. She wasn't one for being told her job, even though it spared this patient a world of hurt.

I was in the hospital for five days. I am the first to admit I am a horrible sick person. I get moody, depressed, and feel like a caged animal. I have so much compassion for those who are bedridden; I can't even imagine.

But I needed to look forward now and keep my spirits high. Up next, the post-surgery pathology report. I was anxious to know the results! I was trying to remain positive.

### *Procedure Day Prayer*

*Heavenly Father, I surrender myself into Your hands.*

*May Your Divine Guidance lead my team of doctors and nurses through my procedure.*

*Surround me with a hundred angels to stand*

*watch*

*over my body and protect my soul.*

*I ask for Your loving presence to be known*

*by all in this medical facility.*

*It is done. It is done. It is done.*

*Thank You.*

## Chapter Six
# Waiting is
# the Hardest Part

**Blog Post: April 8, 2013**

Feels so good to be home and sleep in my own bed. Well, at least until I need to get out of said bed. I didn't realize how many stomach muscles were cut during laparoscopic surgery until I need to use them! And God forbid I need to cough because, at that point, I'm fairly certain the stitches holding my intestines together will rupture, rendering me lifeless. Yeah, I am feeling whiny today, if you haven't noticed.

I have my post-surgery follow-up scheduled for Thursday. I left a message for Dr. N. to call me with the pathology results.

Tick-tock.

It's now past five o'clock. The voice in my head kicks into high gear.

The jabbering won't stop."*He isn't returning your call because he's trying to stall until your appointment on Thursday. Doctors like to deliver bad news in person, you know!*

I can't wait for this to all be over. The weird thing is, today is the first time I feel like the voice is right. I have a strong sense Dr. N. really is avoiding me.

❀ ❀ ❀ ❀ ❀

**Blog Post: April 9, 2013**

First thing in the morning, I call and leave a message for Dr. N. to call me. I want my pathology results.

Tick-tock.

Around 2p.m., I call again. "Please have someone call me with the results from my pathology report." Pretty sure I sound desperate. But hey, if desperate gets me a call back, then I'm all for it!

Around 3:30, my phone rings. I see the caller ID. My heart falls to my stomach. My stomach sinks to my knees. It's Dr. N. He starts talking about the polyp and the part of the colon he removed. The whole time, I am certain there is a "but" coming. He proceeds to tell me how my intestine looked good and the cancer didn't work it's way through the intestinal wall, **_BUT..._**

The cancer did move outside of the colon and was found in two of the fifteen surrounding lymph nodes. He said we'd discuss this in detail at our appointment on Thursday, which is good because my mind was going into shut-down mode. I had read enough about cancer to know spreading to the lymph nodes is a very bad thing, even if it is only two lymph nodes. I liken cancer cells to cockroaches: where there are two, there are *two thousand.*

Cancer is now on the move in my body. Tick-tock.

❦ ❦ ❦ ❦ ❦

## Blog Post: April 10, 2013

I think I slept three hours last night. Why, why does this keep happening? I want off this emotional roller coaster. Stop the ride; I demand my money back!

We are no longer talking about slicing and dicing Linda open so she can be done with cancer and move on with her life. We are entering the twilight zone. At this point, it's a matter of life or death. Okay, perhaps I am being a bit overly dramatic, but if you have never heard your name married to the word cancer, you have NO idea what I'm talking about. Even if you've heard a loved one's name with the word cancer, it's still *not* the same. Call me conceited, but this is now an issue of MY mortality.

I am not insane. I know I will die one day— preferably at a ripe old age after I attend my grandchildren's weddings and hold a few great-grandchildren in my arms. Somehow, being told I have cancer makes all those dreams quickly wash away, and I begin to wonder if I'll even be here next year. My mortality is staring me in the face, taunting me…"So, whacha gonna do now, bitch?"

What am I gonna do now? The obvious answer is FIGHT LIKE HELL. How can I not? That is what everyone expects of me. It's not that I don't want to, but I feel so defeated, and it's only just begun.

❀ ❀ ❀ ❀ ❀

## Blog Post: April 11, 2013

Today is my post-surgery follow-up. This is the appointment where I find out how my life will be changing since I STILL have cancer.

Dr. N. explains how the cancer cells can start moving through the colon wall and easily pop out through the bloodstream, which is how they get into the lymph nodes. Cancer cells are rogue; they don't follow the laws and logic normal cells follow. Cancer cells like to multiply quickly with no rules, rhyme, or reason.

My next step is to meet with an oncologist and discuss my stage and cancer treatment. Dr. N. recommends the oncologist who treated his wife. I think to myself, *Dang, even these doctors and their families can't escape fucking cancer.*

I had been thrown the biggest sucker punch imaginable. I could barely breathe. Was I riding the merry-go-round from hell, or was I stuck in a nightmare? If so, maybe I could wake myself up?

At some point, this all had to stop, right? Or was it going to stop with my life ending? Fear was back like a sociopathic stalker. Fear had full-on engulfed me now.

Fear is a monster. It will convince you that the ugly

future you imagine is most certainly going to come true. If only I had that hindsight and awareness that fear is best described in this perfect acronym, **F**alse **E**vidence **A**ppearing **R**eal.

I licked my wounds again. Sat in my bucket of tears for a day or two and then decided I needed to pull myself together so I could sort out my next steps. Was I going to be the kind of person who throws in the towel, or was I a fighter who keeps moving forward and never looking back?

Clearly, the majority of us want to be the fighter. Being the fighter means you need to tap into those driving forces that will infuse you with the willpower to keep moving in the direction of positive hope for your future. I certainly had many: my blossoming new relationship with a loving man, my children, my desire to see how my children's lives will unfold in the future, my cat, and my deep inner knowing that I still had a purpose to fulfill on this earth.

Armed only with the awareness that I held at this time in my life, I decided to meet with the oncologist and hear what he had to say. I desperately wanted to live. I had so much life left to experience and even more to live for.

### *Meditation of Peace*

Center. Take deep, slow breaths, once you feel your body slow down, repeat the following:

*"My body is at peace.*

*My mind is at peace.*
*My soul is at peace.*
*I drink love into my body.*
*I encapsulate Source Light within every cell of*
*my being.*
*I am not my thoughts.*
*I am strong.*
*I am healed.*
*I am healthy."*
Continue to breathe.

This is a wonderful mantra to carry with you when you feel the overthinking or panic setting in.

## Chapter Seven
# Oncologist Visit

**Blog Post: April 12, 2013**

I waste no time getting an appointment with the oncologist. I've spent time doing research and have learned a lot and gotten very confused and frustrated a lot, too. I am so overwhelmed I break down in tears trying to sort through it all. I eventually concede and decide I'm going to stop overthinking this and just take it all day by day. I will attempt to go with the flow as the information comes to me.

My oncologist is very thorough. He reviews the pathology reports and discusses everything in great detail. He tells me the cells in the cancerous polyp are the same cells found in the lymph nodes—a small relief for me, knowing the cancer didn't come from another place in my body. He goes on to explain when cancer hits the lymph nodes, it puts me automatically at stage three. I think, stage three… that is three of four!?! WTF! The doc explains that I'll need treatment for three days every two weeks for the next six months. Great, this year is pretty much shot!

The next thing I need to do is get a Venus Access Port installed in my chest. Dr. N.'s office can do that procedure at the Surgery Center. That way, the chemo will get plugged in and funneled through the port. Apparently, all that poking and prodding during chemo treatment will ruin the veins in my arms.

The good news to come out of this, if that is even possible, is I won't lose my hair. The oncologist says it will "thin" but shouldn't fall out. I question what a man considers thinning hair, this may not be in line with what a woman considers thinning. Hmmm. At least my pal and stylist, Erin, has my back and scalp. I know she'll help me through any hair crisis!

I tell the oncologist that I want the weekend to think about everything we discussed, and I'll get back to him next week. He assures me that my age and good health makes me a great candidate to come out on the other side of this treatment cancer-free and live a long life.

Greg and I leave the office and without saying a word to one another. We both know damn well that I'll get the treatment. We reunited three years ago with the idea that we will spend the next thirty to forty years together, enjoying one another and our life as much as possible! I'm not about to let him down!

I don't recommend overthinking to anyone. I was in overthink mode on this chemo. The only thing overthinking accomplishes is getting you spun up into a deeper state of fear. And we already gave enough attention to fear in the last couple of chapters. Overthinking is really just jumping ahead and projecting what the future "might" hold. But staying in the "now" was not a part of my knowledge base at the time.

The idea of pumping a cocktail of poison into my body that was still fighting off random cancer cells was unimaginable. But I didn't know anything else. I hadn't thought to study up on alternative treatments, so it wasn't a part of my wheelhouse at this point in my life. I was too scared to not take chemo treatment; I was programmed into believing that is "just what people who have cancer do." So I signed myself up.

For me, this is another situation where hindsight and now my deeper spiritual existence comes into play. Understanding what I inherently know and having my strong spiritual connection to God, my guides and angels, I believe I would reject chemo if I held this knowledge a decade ago. But since I don't have a time machine to go back and see, nor do I wish to relive this experience, we will never know with a hundred percent certainty.

The point I am trying to make is that you, or anyone in a life-threatening situation, will make the choices they need to make based on the knowledge their soul carries at that moment in time. You can't fault yourself or another for those decisions. The saying goes, "You're only as good as the information you're given"; thus, if your place of awareness or lack of awareness is that of "do what the doctor says," then you will. That is where I was.

Now, I am in a place of understanding that doctors are human, just like me. They have schooling, which gives them a knowledge base I do not have; however, it is a Western medicine knowledge base. I am aware there is also Eastern medicine, which has been practiced and healing humans for thousands of years. I am also now aware that there are metaphysical and quantum-based modalities such as Reiki, light therapy, and other types of energy healing modalities available. And I have learned that each individual holds a particular frequency. These frequencies (or vibrations) carry a positive or negative charge. The vibration or frequency you carry has a lot to do with your well-being, too.

If I was told I had cancer today, would I go about it differently? I believe I would. But I also believe *now* that I am destined to live a long, healthy life. Back then, I didn't carry a positive outlook. I was unhappy. I searched for happiness outside of myself. I had carried many regrets. I held repressed anger from many lifetimes. All of these are a formula for creating discordant energy centers in the body. I believe if you carry discordant energy long enough, it will manifest in cancer or other <u>dis</u>-ease. This, in itself, is a subject for another book. There are many knowledgeable writers out there who have written books on this subject if you choose to learn more about this. I merely share with you my thoughts and level of awareness at this point in my journey.

### *Prayer for Decision-Making*

*Dearest Holy Mother Mary,*
*Open my heart to see that path before me*
*with wisdom and clarity.*
*Lead me on this journey.*
*Hold me in the Divine Womb of Creation*
*so the decision I make for my health,*
*Bringing forth the highest and best outcome.*
*May your love serve as*
*a guiding light on my journey.*
*In God's name, it is done.*

## Chapter Eight
# Chemo Prep: The Daze Leading Up to Treatment

**Blog Post: April 14, 2013**

Anti-Social or Social Media? Today, on social media, I posted the following status regarding my cancer.

*"OK, so I'm just gonna rip the band-aid off and put it out there...*

*Went to the doc and the oncologist last week. I found out that I have stage 3 colon cancer. Yes, as in three out of four stages. Good, absolutely not. Fixable, hell to the YES! What now, you say? Once I heal from surgery, I start six months of chemotherapy. After that, my plan is to be 100% cancer-free! Damn good plan, I say!"*

Some may look at this as a social media faux pas. Others might look at it with mild disdain, thinking that the information is way too personal to share in such a broad-based manner. But to me, it's called SOCIAL media for a reason.

By definition:

Social: An informal social gathering, esp. one organized by the members of a particular group: "a church social."

Media: The main means of mass communication regarded collectively: "the campaign won media attention."

Today, I am doing just that, communicating information to everyone in my chosen group. How else am I going to tell over 100 of my friends, family, and close acquaintances that I need to go through chemotherapy? I'm feeling overwhelmed as it is; I certainly can't imagine making that many phone calls or writing that many emails.

As the day progresses, I watch the benefit of my raw honesty unfold. The outpouring of love and encouragement from everyone washes over me like a tsunami. I am deeply touched and left speechless. I have always considered myself a connoisseur of inherently good people. And in recent years, I've even done some purging by abandoning those who wish to bring negativity and hate into my life. Sadly, it took me forty-odd years to realize you <u>can</u> break up with friends, even family, if they aren't good for you. So, as difficult as it is to throw myself out there, I'm glad I am because it's the high-octane fuel driving me to beat this thing.

❀ ❀ ❀ ❀ ❀

## Blog Post: April 17, 2013

Tatt me up before I go, go!

Tattoos. You love 'em, or you hate 'em. I don't believe there is an in-between.

I'm a tatted girl from way back. I got my first tattoo sometime around 1998 or '99. My second tattoo was in 2002, shortly after my mother passed away. And my third was in 2011, during a trip to Miami for my daughter's 18th birthday.

For the past two years, I've been thinking about my fourth tattoo. I know I want a lotus flower, I just don't know where I'd put it on my body or how I'd want it to look.

As I get closer to my impending chemotherapy, I know I'm going to need something symbolic that I can focus on to get me through the process. The lotus tattoo is the first thing that comes to mind. The lotus flower

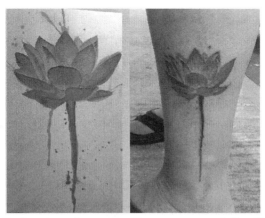

L: drawing of my tattoo R: tattoo on my left calf

symbolizes rising from a dark place into beauty and rebirth, as this is precisely how a lotus flower grows. Lotus flowers bloom directly out of muddy and murky waters and produce beautiful colored blossoms.

I meet with my tattoo artist, Eddie. I decide I want it to look like a watercolor painting. After doing research online we can't find any tattoo examples that are representative of what I want. Being the awesome artist that he is, Eddie goes out and buys watercolor paints so he can make my tattoo from scratch!

❀ ❀ ❀ ❀ ❀

## Blog Post: April 18, 2013

I am in a dark & twisty place today. Everyone is getting under my skin, even my BFFs. I have friends that only want to talk about my cancer. A friend warns me about eating out while I'm off work and recovering from my surgery. I have a friend that wants to dote over me as if I'm made of eggshells. Another who asks every day when my chemo will start. I have friends that constantly tell me "stay positive" to the point where I want to implode! PLEASE, don't get me wrong—I cherish all my friends immensely, and I do feel like the biggest asshole on the planet for feeling this way, but I can't help it! I chalk it up to stress.

In all fairness, I can't say I know how to treat a friend with cancer, either. When my BFF, Judi, was dying of colon cancer, I made a point to let her update me on her treatment, and then I would fill the rest of our conversation with humorous anecdotal blather. I would make sure and discuss the future, telling her how I was making plans to visit her real soon. Sadly, her untimely death came before I made it out to Colorado to see her. A painful regret I'll carry with me forever. ANYHOW, enough of my mournful reminiscing. After all these years, Judi remains in my heart and is always on my mind. I'm certain she knows that, too.

ꙮ ꙮ ꙮ ꙮ ꙮ

## Blog Post: April 19, 2013

A New Port—Full Sail Ahead.

Today is port installation day. I wonder if they have a Hallmark card for that? I can't say I'm looking forward to going back to the Surgery Center, even though they treat me well. I know I promised myself I'm just going to *keep moving forward*, *go through the motions*, and continue to take it *one day at a time*. I'm guessing it is times like these when all those wonderful clichés get invented.

Dr. N. stops by to tell me the procedure takes only ten to fifteen minutes; however, from the time I enter the operating room to the time I exit is a little over an hour. The anesthesiologist injects the magical twilight drug into my IV, and I am out before I even leave the holding area.

Once I wake up, I notice I have this huge bandage on my chest. I get queasy at the thought of what is underneath. I'm achy and sore and can feel the foreign object inside me with every move I make.

As Greg drives me home, I stare out the window and wonder how I'm going to make peace with this new chapter in my life.

The myriad of emotions, feelings, and frustrations for a person going through cancer is overwhelming at times. I could be feeling upbeat one day and a couple hours later seeing only doom and gloom in my future.

For caregivers, family, and other loved ones of those going through cancer, it is important to not take what they say personally. In fact, you should *never* take what another person says personally. People act or react from their own personal feelings or trauma.

There is a great book called *The Four Agreements* (there is actually a fifth agreement now) by Don Miguel Ruiz. It's a fabulous book based on ancient Toltec wisdom that will lead you to personal freedom. The book is a code of conduct that frees one from self-limiting beliefs.

Don Miguel Ruiz believes if you follow these four agreements, your life will markedly improve. 1. Be impeccable with your word. 2. Don't take anything personally. 3. Don't make assumptions. 4. Always do your best. And the new fifth agreement: Be skeptical, but learn to listen.

The people who stood by me and supported me

during this journey were the lifeblood I needed in order to see myself coming out on the other side of the Big C. As a friend or caregiver of a person going through cancer, I would suggest that you find caring ways to express your love for them, as well as help distract them from their constant cancer thoughts. Buy mindless magazines or movies, talk about funny anecdotal things you've experienced lately, buy a trashy novel or Sci-Fi book for them to read.

I wish I had knowledge of Don Miguel's ancient Toltec wisdom when I was going through my cancer year. I look back on my blog posts now and see a much less evolved and semiconscious Linda. I don't hold judgment over that version of me; she only did what she knew at the time. In fact, I can clearly see the vast expansion and soul growth, both in my spiritual beliefs and conscious awareness. It feels good to see progress. I still fall into a smidgen of regret sometimes, wishing I had this knowledge decades ago, but then I remember that my soul needed this experience so I could learn this wonderfully expansive lesson and feel this exponential growth during my human experience.

### *Prayer of Thanks for Caregivers*

*It is with deep gratitude that I call forth the Angels of God.*

*Surround my caregiver with Your Divine Love.*

*Hold them in strength and grace*

*as they offer up themselves in service*

*to my healing and well-being.*

*May my deep reverence for their compassion be evident.*

*May their offerings be expressed in grace and ease.*

*May their unwavering service be the beacon through which they realize their own inner light.*

*Hold these caregivers in Your sanctimonious praise.*

*As through the Glory of His Angels,*

*all is possible,*

*all will be exalted.*

## Chapter Nine
# Hey, Bartender, Pass Me One of Those Chemo Cocktails

**Blog Post: April 29, 2013**

Today is a big day for two reasons. First reason: it's the day I go back to work after being off for four weeks. Second reason: it's my "chemo teach," a scary yet necessary part of my cancer journey.

I arrive at work at 8 a.m. feeling strange, like I really don't belong. I slink quietly down the hall to my office. But as soon as I open the door, it was like I just returned after a long weekend. The familiarity and the pile of *git'er done* assignments gave levity to my step. I long to feel preoccupied, and now my wish is granted.

The second part of the day is getting schooled on how my chemo will go down. Greg and I meet with Barbara, a nurse that looks to be in her mid-fifties or so. She gives it to me straight. She introduces me to my new friends, Eloxatin, Fluorouracil (otherwise known as "5-FU," for real! I'm not making that up), and their trusty sidekick, Leucovarin. She rattles off a laundry list of nasty-ass side effects: numbness in my hands & feet, thinning hair, mouth sores, constipation, diarrhea, fatigue, loss of appetite, sensitivity to light, taste changes, discoloration along veins where the medication is given, low blood counts, and nail discoloration or loss. The strangest side effect that she says is common in almost all patients is the inability to drink or touch anything cold. If you drink cold liquids, it feels like you're swallowing razor blades; if you touch anything cold, it feels like you're being stabbed with knives. She suggests wearing gloves if I need to retrieve anything from the freezer or fridge. I think to myself, *What the hell do people up north do if they need treatment in the winter?* The weirdness of it all starts to get to me, and I fight back tears.

Barbara continues outlining procedures: what to bring to chemo, what blood tests will be done at the beginning of each round. She tells me I need to avoid buffets and salad bars, crowded places, small children, and the sun, if possible (or wear a good SPF). No showers on chemo days unless I have a handheld shower nozzle so I can avoid getting the port wet. The list goes on and on, and my brain begins to tune her out as I start making a mental list off of all the things I can't do this year.

Then, she opens the floor for questions. Greg and I look at each other dumbfounded. She can sense we're clueless, so she tries to pull questions out of us.

"Who cooks in your house?"

Again, we are both like Dumb and Dumber, unsure how to answer.

Finally, I say, "I used to cook more, but not much lately. And Greg is really good at grilling."

Barbara looks at Greg and says, "Okay, you're going to have to take over cooking duties. Know that most days, she may not want to eat, but try to give her something. And if she asks for something, and by the time you make it and bring it to her, she doesn't want it, don't get mad, just put it away for a while, and she may eat it later."

Then she says, "What about sex?"

Say WHHHHHAAAAAAAAT??!! I look at Barbara and say, "Um, are you asking if we have sex, like sex, plan on sex, or all of the above? And if you're getting ready to tell me there is NO sex during chemo, then you can watch me walk out that door right now, and you'll never see me again."

She chuckles, "No, you can have sex, but you may not feel up to it because you'll be so exhausted." She looks at Greg and says, "So you'll need to be patient and understanding."

Greg replies, "Between the surgery and the port, she has so many holes in her I'm afraid I'll hurt her."

"Well, you only need one hole, honey!" she quipped.

Way to go, Nurse Barbara! You the (wo)man!

My first chemo appointment is a week from today.

Hopefully, they keep me this entertained for the next six months.

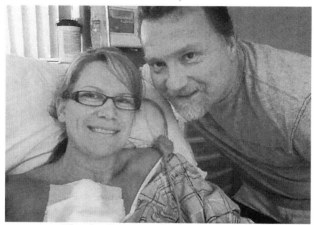

*The day I got my chemo port installed –*
*the port provides a more efficient way to deliver the cocktail*
*and saves your veins from repetitive trauma.*

This chemotherapy appointment made this theatrical production full of twists and turns of uncertainty all too real. I was no longer watching myself act out a bit part, I was now the star. Intermission is over. My nemesis, colon cancer, enters, stage three. My second act is now underway.

As I reflect back, I see my year of cancer truly was the beginning of my second act. The love of my life came in at the end of the first act to see me through to the end of this production.

As mentioned earlier, Greg and I were high school

sweethearts. We had an on-again, off-again relationship in our early years. What inevitably would always split us apart was Greg's desire to be off again so that he could spend time with his friends, skipping school and partying. I much prefer the on-again parts of having a boyfriend.

Between the ages of sixteen and twenty-one, we struggled to find a way to make it work. There was this underlying camaraderie because of the way we were both raised. We were products of divorce, living with single parents. Our mothers raised us more like feral cats than like children. We were each left to our own devices. This made us a perfect match for one another.

The love part for us was a bit more challenging. It wasn't just the way we were raised and our free-spirited personalities that drew us together; there was this deep, underlying, unspoken knowledge that we had done this together many times before. I am a believer in reincarnation. I think the jury is still out for Greg. Either way, we both feel the deep attraction at the soul level. When Greg told his brother we were getting back together, the first thing his brother said was, " That's great. It always felt like you two had some unfinished business." We may not understand it, but we both feel that too.

As we entered into this renewed relationship almost thirty years later, we both knew we needed to address traumas from our previous life. We also knew talk therapy would be a benefit. But, like weeds, traumas have a way of creeping back in unless you dig way down deep and remove them at the roots. We had been dealing with them the first couple of years, but now we needed to table all that. Cancer was a far more formidable monster than we had ever encountered, and to exterminate it, we had to present a united front.

I am so grateful for the way this all aligned. It may be hard for some of you to understand how one can be grateful for their cancer, but many times, I have witnessed the perfection of how this scenario was orchestrated. If I would've been in my previous marriage, I likely would've just given up and resigned myself to checking out. But I had Greg in my life now, someone my heart had been longing for during our years apart. I wasn't about to let this next chapter end abruptly. Like Greg's brother said, we had unfinished business to attend to.

Admittedly, it is hard for me to look back on the previous blog post discussing my chemotherapy. I know I made the best decision, based on my level of consciousness at the time; however, through the crystal-clear lens of hindsight, plus knowing what I know now, if I was presented with this today, I would do things very differently.

And I will say it for those who need this clarity and confirmation: I am not an expert, I am not a medical professional; I am simply an individual who now has a larger knowledge base and a higher consciousness than I had upon entering into this cancer journey. The vantage point changes EVERYTHING.

Make no mistake about it: chemotherapy is toxic. It is a poison—at least, this is how I would describe it. Maybe your medical practitioner sees it differently. The thing is, I still suffer the consequences of the drugs that I used during chemotherapy. The bottoms of my feet are numb from neuropathy; it contributes to the restless leg syndrome that I feel during the night. Fortunately, I have been able to alleviate that pain with a grounding sheet on my bed. Chemo also contributed to my need for cataract surgery at age fifty-seven. Prolonged use of steroids, which was part of my chemo cocktail, is never a good idea. Those are just a couple of the issues that I deal with today.

What I'm saying is, if you are at a place where you were guided to read this book, then perhaps your consciousness is at a higher level than mine was when I entered into this journey. Again, if I could go back and do it all again, I would do some heavy research into the drugs they wanted to pump into my body. I also would have stopped my treatments at the very first sign of neuropathy creeping into my feet. Instead, I felt like I needed to "tough it out" and get all of them in and get to the end.

But, upon further review, from my now thirty-thousand-foot view, I can see that every single part, down to the finest detail, was also perfectly orchestrated to lead me down the path that I am on now. So perhaps it wasn't the idea that I wasn't as conscious then as I am now; perhaps it's the script that I agreed to adhere to when my soul came to experience this lifetime. I know these are very grandiose, abstract ideas, but this is also the place that I have been led to throughout my journey as my spiritual heart and consciousness have expanded exponentially over the years.

I speak only from my personal perspective, but coming out on the other side of a stage-three cancer diagnosis will forever change you. And isn't that what most of us are looking for, anyway? We are all in search of the thing that will totally light us up. The experience that will elevate us out of our misery and into a space of joy. I don't live a perfect life, and Greg and I still have challenges to work through, but overall, from that thirty-thousand-foot view, we have a damn good life! And although it seems like it all happened by chance, it really happened because we followed that well-written script that we were given before we came to this planet of amnesia. A planet of duality, where you are driven to live amongst the good and the bad, learning to observe without triggers, without attachment. And I am just grazing the surface of what this place is all about.

### *Meditation to Expand Awareness*

*Breathe in slow and deep, all the way down the body to your root chakra.*

*Feel your Earth Star chakra below you in the ground as your breath sinks deep into the earth below you. Connect to that Earth Star chakra, anchoring it in.*

*Pull the breath up, high into your head, and through your crown. Feel your connection to your Soul chakra, which resides roughly six inches above your head. Feel into that space above your head and anchor in.*

*As you breathe, feel your breath move down into the Earth Star chakra and then up again through each of your body's chakra points (Root - Sacral - Solar Plexus, Heart - Throat - Third Eye - Crown ) and up to your Soul chakra. And then down again.*

*Bring your awareness through each chakra point and the part of the body in which it resides. Focus only on the breath and the movement up and down through your body.*

*Cycle through the up-and-down breath for seven cycles.*

Once you complete the seven cycles, bring the breath back into its normal rhythm. Sit in quiet contemplation. Note how your body feels. This is a wonderful opportunity to journal the sensations and feelings that come through.

## Chapter Ten
# God & Cancer

**Blog Post: May 2, 2013**

I may have mentioned that I like to overthink things. I'm not sure if that's an A.D.D. trait or what. On my drive to work, I wondered why I got cancer. There must be some deeper meaning in all this.

I was raised Catholic; however, I am not a practicing Catholic. I haven't totally denounced my upbringing, but through the years, I have grown to consider myself more of a spiritual person than a religious one. I don't believe one religion is better than another. In fact, I tend to embrace aspects from many religions, my own spiritual buffet, if you will. I do believe in only one God; that is a given.

I also have this inherent certainty that God does not give us more than we can handle. So, for some reason, God feels I can handle my cancer and the impending chemotherapy. With that in mind, I wonder why I got cancer in the first place, and I'm guessing that everyone who gets cancer thinks the same thing. This brings me to the second part of my belief: I am supposed to learn an important lesson from my cancer journey. I create daily laundry lists in my head of the possible lessons to learn.

In turn, I wonder if I manifested this in my own life. Is it the emotional baggage I've carried around since childhood? Could it be the stress of a highly-charged marriage and an overly demanding career that finally caught up with me? Or is it really just the luck of the draw in a genetic poker game?

As you can see, this overthinking is a bitch that I need to kick to the curb and leave along the roadside to fend for herself. My lesson today? Start meditating and clear these thoughts out of my head.

As I reflect back, I realize now that this became the pivotal point in my spiritual journey. I wondered why God would let His children suffer. I knew my God is not a vengeful and fearful one, so there has to be a purpose why many lead lives of suffering.

If God indeed does not give us more than we can handle, then my Creator knows I am strong enough to get through this. In my soul, I know this is not going to be my exit point from this planet. This is where I step into a state of awareness that my life needed some big changes. Changes that would lead to a long and healthy life. Cancer is not going to seal my fate.

As I moved through the next decade of my life, my beliefs began to morph. I spent my time searching for answers. What is my purpose? Clearly, I had one, or I wouldn't still be here. The Source, our Creator, surely doesn't assign us these human travesties, so why do they exist?

There are some deep concepts I discovered through meditation, learning about awakening and spirituality, that resonate as truths for me now. These truths fall in line with my beliefs on reincarnation as well.

I believe that our souls are eternal. They choose the lessons and experiences we wish to have on this planet. In every incarnation, we collaborate with other souls, playing each other's good guys and villains, in order to create your soul's desired human experience. All the while we are having this experience, we are also carrying out a mission. Your mission is your life's purpose, what you came here to unfold, create, and manifest.

Each soul is an intricate cog in the wheel called planet Earth. The Earth is an important part of this galaxy: she is also playing a role. Our galaxy depends on our Earth's evolution and the people who inhabit her. That greater purpose I have yet to determine, but I have some ideas. I'll save those thoughts for another book.

We are all part of an intricate tapestry, no thread better or worse than another. The darkness and the light coexist to create the tapestry's design. Each is needed. Each is important.

These are some of the truths you may begin to unfold when you are in the midst of a deep dive during your cancer journey.

Please know I am not sharing all this with you because I feel you need to believe as I do; we each have our own unique path. However, should you be feeling curious and are open-minded, you may want to explore ideas like this for yourself.

Humans are not stagnant creatures; we are ever-evolving beings of light. We embody an everlasting soul that lives in this meat suit as we carry out our human experience. How will you carry out the rest of *yours*?

### *Prayer of Eternal Light*

*Creator of All that Is,*

*I am a conduit for Your Eternal Light.*

*Guide me through my healing with expanded awareness.*

*Show me the purpose of my journey so that I may heal.*

*Reveal my soul's true path so that I may course-correct.*

*Open my eyes to any unseen discord in my life.*

*Enliven my heart with the courage to step into my authentic self.*

*I will carry Your Eternal Light as I fully step into the life my BEing is here to experience.*

## Chapter Eleven
# Finding My Spiritual Nature

**Blog Post: May 31, 2013**

When faced with your own mortality, one starts to look at the world differently. Sure, we're all gonna die one day, but when the possibility of dying becomes YOUR reality, it's then, and only then, that you stop and take pause. Sure there are a few of you who have mastered the art of being centered, so much so that you joyously bound through life, rolling with the punches, knowing that each day is a gift, and that's why it's called the present. I envy you. Me, I seem to haphazardly tumble through life, aimlessly tending to whatever is set in front of me, dwelling on the past and worrying about the future. I'm never quite able to unwrap the elusive "present." Sure, I see it sitting there. And I want it bad. But as much as I want it, I tend to get wrapped up in the drama that seems to surround my life.

I don't fancy myself a drama queen. However, some may argue, and you know who you are, that perhaps I create all the drama that surrounds me. To that, I say most definitely not. I know people (you know who you are) who love to swirl in a sea of drama. If drama isn't happening, they feel the need to create their own. Somehow, I seem to attract these people like flies, and therein lies the problem. Knowing this about myself, through the years, I have slowly started eliminating these drama queens and kings from my life. That was my first step.

The second step is to start surrounding myself with loving, caring people who have that thing that I want. People who live in the now. Those who choose inner peace over outward materialism. I can no longer tolerate being around those who are driven by money, power, and greed. Not that I could ever handle that type of personality, but in the past took the passive approach, I made excuses for that type of behavior, and looked the other way, somehow justifying their shallowness.

Third, I need to practice being the type of person I want to meet. It sounds silly, like I'm inexperienced on how to be myself. The truth is we're all a work in progress, that is the beauty of being human. We're all like a clay sculpture that is never quite complete. Our family, our life experiences, both past and present, our jobs, and the people we come in contact with every day all play a part in molding our clay.

Part of my studies on how to become the me I want to be include meditation. You would think that is a simple enough task, however, my personality tends to be the opposite of everything that meditation represents. I'm an overthinker, I am A.D.D., I can't sit still, I can't leave things undone, I guess I'm a bit anal retentive. These are not the best traits for someone who wishes to meditate and be *in the now*. The good news is, I know this about myself, so I'm halfway there!

Last year, Greg and I took a class on how to meditate. Again, sounds silly that we need a class on how to sit still and clear our minds. I've tried meditation on my own, on and off, for years and never could figure out how to shut off my brain. So, this class was a great way for both of us to learn techniques. It was one hour a week, for four weeks. Every week when I left meditation class I felt this high. My whole body was like Jello. My mind was at peace. Sadly, I couldn't retain that feeling for more than an hour or so after class. Reality is a cold, cruel bitch, and she came knocking on my door with a baseball bat, making sure I snapped out of it. I always thought if I could just push myself into meditation for a mere fifteen minutes a day, I'd become a better person and soon learn to push that bitch, reality, back out the door.

Now that I've had mortality rattle my cage, I've sharpened my focus on creating zen moments in my life and ultimately finding my bliss. I know it will take baby steps. I also know it will require discipline and practice. Today I've started putting the process into motion by designing a meditative healing garden.

During recovery from my colon resection surgery and throughout my first two cycles of chemotherapy, I have found that spending time in my screen porch is very relaxing. Sitting under the ceiling fans, gazing out at the two giant oaks and all the little critters that call them home, is quite soothing. However, this one corner of the yard, to the left of my porch, was a big ol' mess of dirt and weeds. I thought it would be great if I could brighten that spot by creating my own healing garden to serve as a source of beauty and serenity on my journey to finding my zen.

And so I did.

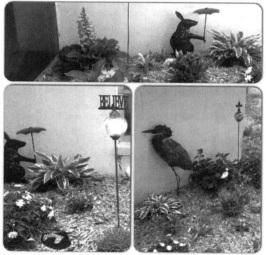

*My zen garden. My tiny corner of serenity as I heal.*

I found this deeply resonant description of zen by Roshi Pat Enkyo O'Hara. "Real Zen is the practice of coming back to the actual right-now-in-this-moment self, coming back to the naturalness, the intimacy, and simplicity of our true nature. Zen practice is not about getting away from our life as it is; it is about getting into our life as it is, with all of its vividness, beauty, hardship, joy, and sorrow. Zen is a path of awakening: awakening to who we really are, and awakening the aspiration to serve others and take responsibility for all of life."

Zen was definitely a quest for my soul during my cancer journey and beyond. Unwittingly, I began my own practice of *zazen* (a seated meditation). I would gaze at my oaks, breathe in my garden, observe nature in the now moment. I quickly found that nature, one of my true loves, was also a place that offered me profound soul healing.

On the days I had my "take home" chemo treatment and was able to stay awake, I would sit on my porch and soak in nature from my backyard. On my chemo off-weeks, I would get out for walks at the 162-acre park across the road from my house.

The true physical healing of nature is incredible. If you walk barefoot on the ground, you can absorb the earth's electrons. This is called "earthing." It's nothing new; I just believe it's gotten lost over the centuries as modern medicine pushed nature's remedies into the background. Combine earthing with forest bathing and sunshine, and you've hit the trifecta of nature's healing power.

For a decade now, I have incorporated nature walks into my daily schedule. It is the way I meditate. I can walk for miles in complete clarity of Spirit. Many times, I will receive messages from my higher self/ my inner knowing that help me gain insights into our world, or I may receive channeled messages from ascended masters or other benevolent beings. Nature is where I pray. Nature is my spiritual fuel. If I don't get out into the woods or among the trees, I get agitated and start to fall into a funk.

When I work with clients in my spiritual practice, I consistently recommend the healing power of nature. The outdoors immediately transports your spirit into a simpler place. The calming presence of the trees, the soothing rhythm of the cicadas, the healing melody of a bird's song, or the elation of capturing a glimpse of a wild deer or fox. One or all of these combined nurture our souls and bring us to a place of nonjudgment in the present moment.

Indigenous tribes across the planet know the healing power of nature. Mother Earth is their home, and they honor her with deep reverence for the gifts she provides.

My spirituality is tied strongly to Gaia, our planet Earth. Her forest is my temple. Her animals are my teachers. Her elements guide me. The stars above her are my ancestors. Her oceans comfort me. Her mountains reveal their ancient wisdom. Her flowers expose her natural beauty. We are nothing without her, and she would be perfectly fine without any of us. She is mother to us all. Respect for her is imperative to our existence.

### *Prayer to Mother Gaia (Mother Earth)*

*Mother Gaia,*

*Thank you for showering resplendent healing energy upon me during this time of suffering.*

*I seek solace within your gifts of the*

*forests, oceans, and mountains.*

*Your warm breeze envelops me with a loving embrace.*

*Your sturdy pines sing songs of harmony as they bend and sway in the wind.*

*The passing butterfly is a gentle reminder of my own transformation.*

*The birds sing glorious songs of joy, harkening the day ahead.*

*I walk barefoot, feeling the mossy softness of your earthly splendor.*

*Your creatures small and mighty are spirited reminders of the beautiful home you've created for us all.*

*For all this, I am forever grateful.*

## Chapter Twelve
# Chemo's Dirty Little Secrets: Part One

**Blog Post: June 4, 2013**

Today is a bad day. I had so much hope when my second cycle went so well, I actually thought I'd be able to breeze through all consecutive cycles the same way. Well, not so much. I liken today to being hit by a Mack Truck. I'm extremely lethargic, yet unable to sleep. I intermittently lose feeling in my hands, and my fingers cramp and contort in ways I can't control on my own. I stumble through sentences, feeling occasional bouts of chemo brain. I feel nauseous even with my anti-nausea medicine. The hot flashes are coming fast and furious, so much so I swear I will spontaneously combust. Blah, blah, blah… I could go on and on but I'd just scare off any readers I've accumulated up to this point!

So what does one do when one is home from work dealing with the backlash of chemotherapy? Why, watch the show *The Big C*, of course! I was sad to see that the final season is only four episodes, however, each one packs a big punch. The whole series was so well written and touched me deeply, more so now than ever before. During the series finale of *The Big C* there is a scene that really resonates with me. It is Cathy's conversation with the priest, rabbi, and Muslim imam (I *think* that is what a Muslim priest is called) when she was at hospice. The imam said, "Your illness is not just to test you, but to test the charity of others. Have you seen generosity and kindness in the people around you? Well, we believe that beauty and the knowledge of that goodness is Allah."....WOW!

Over the past two months I have been humbled by the generosity of friends both near and far. As I said in an earlier post, I get cards, gifts, and well wishes via emails or posts every day. To me it's not the material objects that give me a rush; it's the fact that for some reason I am blessed to be surrounded by so many people who genuinely care about me. Pre-cancer Linda never sat and truly considered that there would be a time when she would feel such a warm embrace from all these smiling faces that she's collected throughout her lifetime. She simply was drawn to those who were likeminded. Cancer Linda is now reminded on a daily basis how blessed she is to have such an amazing circle of friends. You share your generosity and kindness with me. The knowledge of that goodness is God. WOW!

I started a wall of cards with all the well wishes I've received via snail mail. The power of the handwritten word on the inside of a Hallmark card still has amazing, heartfelt power. Don't get me wrong: it doesn't in any way diminish the other well wishes I've received electronically; those are also a thing of beauty that I cherish! The cool thing about my wall of cards is that it serves as my daily visual reminder that I am not in this alone. Each of those cards represents all the people that are on my side, friends who truly care and are rooting for me to kick cancer's ass! Again, the goodness that is God.

In the words of *The Big C's* Cathy Jamison, LUCKY ME....LUCKY ME.

❦ ❦ ❦ ❦ ❦

**Blog Post: June 9, 2013**

Another 4 a.m. wake-up call. Sleep doesn't come easy for me. For well over a decade now, I've been plagued by sleeplessness. The vicious cycle began thirteen years ago when my son Noah was born, or, as I call him, my naughty non-sleeper. It took him several *YEARS* to sleep through the night, and at that point, I began shifting into my job stress-TMJ-teeth grinding phase. I finally corrected that sleeping disorder by finding a new job. It wasn't long and my sleeplessness shifted into the deteriorating marriage-teenage children-sole provider stress type of sleeplessness. Which soon gave way to the divorce—heavily burdened by related financial strains-single parenting-sleeplessness. All of which circles around to where I am now with my job stress-family worries-changing dynamics of my personal relationships-chemo ridden sleeplessness cycle, otherwise known as my Midnight Malaise Period.

I'm slowly learning to make the best of my sleepless times. SLOWLY. I admit that the hypnotic lure of social media can easily suck me in at 2 a.m. Sure, I try to conceal my addiction, iPhone in hand, covers drawn over my head. Even in my self-aware, electronically addictive state, I know this isn't giving me any solace long term. But it is a process. I'll slowly work to exchange my online preoccupation for something more substantial. Scout's honor!

However, some nights when my head is wrought with worry, I take to my email and correspond with my Angel, Lee. She is a blessing. Just knowing that at any given time I can reach out to her, no matter what my circumstance, is comforting. Not only is she there, she gets it. Truly gets IT. There seems to be an intuitive bond between those who have walked the hot coals of cancer treatment. A brethren or sisterhood of sorts that has this magical handbook to help us newbies work through the process. For instance, the other day, or I should say, late night at 1 am, I reached out to my Angel Lee just to touch base. I knew she just spent a long weekend with her husband in Rhode Island, celebrating their nineteenth wedding anniversary

AND the one-year anniversary of her last colon cancer treatment—two fabulous milestones! I was curious to hear how it went, since at this point in my treatment, I really do enjoy living vicariously through others!

Lee updates me on her fabulous weekend. And without knowing my inner struggles or perhaps *all-knowing* of my inner struggles, she offers me a bit of unsolicited sentiment to chew on. It's no secret that big, life-changing circumstances alter who we are and how we perceive the world around us, forever. The part that can be hard to swallow is how those life-changing events can also alter our relationships with others. As any good angel would, Lee clearly sensed this struggle with me as she offered me the following perspective:

*My friend Gary, a lymphoma survivor, introduced me to Imerman Angels, and we constantly talk about being blessed. Sounds strange that such a horrible illness could be a blessing, but it truly changes you. No matter what type of person you were, you'll never be the same......but in a great way. The struggle strengthens you. The pain makes you enjoy the pain-free time so much more. You'll appreciate your friends and family that have stepped up, especially the ones you never expected to. With that also comes disappointment in the ones that you thought would, but that changes YOU. I will never walk away from anyone for any reason. Small needs are just as important as big ones.*

As I lay here wide awake at 4 a.m. during my shittiest week of chemo thus far, I still manage to feel blessed. I am incredibly humbled at the thoughtfulness of family and friends who continually reach out to me with love, support, and prayers. In turn, I am seeking understanding as I part ways with those who do not have the capacity to travel on this journey with me, learning that it is their burden to contend with, not mine. I thank God every day that I have this solid rock of a man by my side, loving me unconditionally, cheering me on, lifting my spirits, and keeping me grounded in reality so I don't slip away into a dark and twisty place. My three children give me purpose and the strength to fight so I can witness their future greatness—big or small, it's all greatness to this Mama!

❀ ❀ ❀ ❀ ❀

## Blog Post: June 18, 2013

Chemotherapy is a bitch. Treatment 3 was really rough on me, and I entered my fourth cycle in a weakened state, my white blood count continually dropping and now hovering below the normal range, which tells me my body is fighting harder and harder to repair after each treatment. My feet are numb, which makes me shuffle around the house like an 85-year-old woman. My fingers won't listen to my brain and seize up when I least expect it (so please forgive any type-o's as I type this with two bent fingers—thank God for the iPhone's talk-to-type feature!). My daily nausea is controlled by drugs that make me loopy. I'll shut up now because I could go on and on with this pity party.

I am grateful for those around me who check in and show their concern, as those little "boosts" help me keep up the fight. I'm slowly coming to the realization that I can't do it all, and for someone like me, who is a people-pleasing perfectionist and planner, that is very difficult to accept. I'm not one to release control and admit I can't make dinner, clean the house, or get out of bed and go to work. It just isn't in my nature. But as my oncologist and chemo nurses tell me, I must. I have to put myself, my health and well-being (physical and mental) FIRST. I know what they're saying is correct, so why is it so hard for me to accept?

Times like this, I am thankful for my angel. Someone who has been there and done that. She is my solace in the middle of the night when I need to vent or my mind is racing with so many unknowns.

I want to share this exchange between my angel and me…then you, too, can see what a shining light she is during this dark time in my life. And to any of my colon cancer friends that I've met in online threads, perhaps you can glean some hope, knowledge, and inspiration from these emails as well.

❀ ❀ ❀ ❀ ❀

**Email from Lee to Linda: 8:56 p.m. on Monday**

Sounds like I had the same regimen you're having. My hands and feet were extremely sensitive. I couldn't touch anything cold, and I always had to wear slippers while at home and usually two pairs of socks when

I went out. Especially bad all four days after each treatment. Any time I stepped outdoors, I had a scarf around my neck, mouth, and nose. Couldn't handle cold.

At night, my legs and feet used to spasm, too. So crazy. I would try to get up and walk it out, but nothing helped.

What are you feeling?

Are you wiped out tonight?

I remember not wanting to eat a thing when I returned from the city. It was almost always a ten-to-twelve-hour day from the time I left my home until I returned. Sometimes, I got very nauseous coming home because we sat in stop-and-go traffic forever.

So many factors made it worse.

Talk soon.

Lee

Sent from my iPhone

❀ ❀ ❀ ❀ ❀

**Email from Linda to Lee: 12:45 a.m. Tuesday**

I'm having atrophy in my hands & feet, plus intermittent numbness in both. The exhaustion is extreme, but the steroids in the chemo keep me waking up. The cold is extreme the first week, but my crazy, frequent hot flashes are offsetting that a lot. Plus, the first bite of food I take each time I try to eat causes incredible pain in the back of my mouth by my glands. I can't eat much as it causes stomach upset, plus I'm just plain crabby about it all... I dread those Mondays now & wonder how I'm going to do it without giving up. I know all my friends are well-meaning by telling me how strong I am, but I don't feel it. I feel angry & weak, like giving up. Greg is very supportive, but I just want to run away like an injured animal & be alone to lick my wounds. I try to find positives, but the first week is always bad & seems to be getting worse. from Linda's iPhone

❀ ❀ ❀ ❀ ❀

**Email from Lee to Linda: 8:02 a.m. Tuesday**

Flat out—it sucks. I get it.

I know everyone around you means well and tries to help, but you still feel alone. You're voluntarily beating the crap out of yourself, always questioning the real need to. I found the need by looking around me. My husband, kids, friends...I wasn't ready to check out or want the C to beat me. Right b4 my fourth treatment was my birthday—I had a complete and total breakdown. Scared to death that I wouldn't celebrate another birthday and petrified of #4 side effects. That was a reality check—make a choice then and there, I thought. I couldn't live in the moment but rather live for tomorrow. Just had to get through the moment. My internist, Dr. A (also a close friend), responded to my daily, even hourly, text messages—usually responding with "tomorrow will be better." That's what I held onto.

I'm here for you today and tomorrow, I promise. I would take it again for you if I could!!! I mean it.
Sent from my iPhone

*ૐ* *ૐ* *ૐ* *ૐ* *ૐ*

**Email from Linda to Lee: 8:41 a.m. Tuesday**

Thank you for your kind words. I've had a couple breakdowns myself. My weakened state seems to get me there pretty quick! Then I do stupid things and add salt to my wounds by reading horrible stories on the internet that say chemo will kill you quicker than the cancer will, not exactly motivational material. :-/

I think I need to find something to look forward to... yes, seeing my kids grow and make a life of their own is a biggie, living many more loving years with the man of my dreams is a biggie too! I need to come up with a short-term incentive that will give me some ME time to look forward to, something I always neglect. Like a trip, a party, or something to celebrate that the biggest part of my battle is over! Not sure what that would be as it seems so far away and I still have other daunting financial and job issues going on behind the scenes that prevent me from actually committing to much of anything. Hence my frustration...

Thank you for listening. It is comforting to have someone there who "gets it."
xoxo
from Linda's iPhone

*ૐ* *ૐ* *ૐ* *ૐ* *ૐ*

**Email from Lee to Linda: 8:02 a.m. Tuesday**

After my 6th we took a few days trip with my brother and his family to Georgia. Airports and planes present a risk, but we rolled the dice. To this day, Dr. A says that helped me so much get thru the rest. It was something to look forward to, and the change of scenery was even more beneficial. Loads of sunscreen and, of course, a wide variety of hats.

We even went horseback riding on the beach—another risk but Dr. A knew the benefits there. The funniest was while we were there, I was getting ready for dinner, went to put my wig on, and forgot my wig cap. My only alternative was my daughter's panties. We were all cracking up as I pranced around the room without the wig. All thru dinner, my niece would have me do the bobblehead to be sure the wig didn't slip. Laughter heals!

Instead of a major blow out party, we planned a big trip for last August. A true celebration for me, Mike, Michael, Mack, and Annie. I started the planning around treatment #8. Kept my brain on a dream. Hawaii-paradise.

If u can, plan a special dinner date or an overnight. (How about a trip to NYC?) 😊 It helps!

Rest rest rest.

Sent from my iPhone

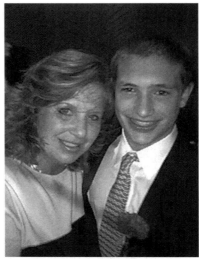

*My angel, Lee with 1 of her 3 children.*

My dear friend, Kelly, turned me on to this amazing organization that assisted a friend of hers through cancer. It is called Immerman Angels. This incredible organization provides free, personalized one-on-one cancer support for cancer fighters, survivors, previvors, and caregivers.

I am one who hesitates to ask for help. Truthfully, I actually don't ask for help. But cancer was so far out of my comfort zone and comprehension that I needed someone in my life who "got it." Sure, I could vent and share with my partner, but how was he to truly understand what I was experiencing? So, I did this uncharacteristic thing and reached out for an angel to assist me. And let me tell you, it was the best decision.

I don't know how I would have managed to get through this cancer journey without Lee. We were perfectly matched. We both had three kids, and we are roughly the same age. We had the same stage of colon cancer. She had the same treatment protocol. So, she knew exactly what I was dealing with during my treatments. What a Godsend!

If I can encourage a cancer patient to do just one thing, it is to ask for help! Do you realize there are people in your life right now that are frozen, they have absolutely no idea what to say or do for you? They are paralyzed with fear. And YOU can be the person to help them overcome that fear. Give them a job! YES! It will be an amazing icebreaker for them and help you more than you can imagine!

Need a couple loads of laundry done? Groceries picked up? A casserole for dinner Tuesday night? The lawn mowed? The kids picked up from soccer practice? All you need to do is shove your crazy pride aside and ASK.

Here's the thing: people like to feel needed. People like to be helpful. By not asking, you are refusing someone who cares about you the opportunity to help.

I look back now and realize how nuts I was for not asking for more help. I had to be supermom, superwoman; I had to ride my type-A personality all the way through cancer treatment. Don't be like me. Ask!

### *Breath Work to Release Pain*

- Get comfortable, lying slightly propped up with pillows or sitting back in a recliner.
- Make sure your head is supported.
- Keep your shoulders down.
- First, exhale, then breathe in through your nose. Your stomach should rise as air enters and lower as you breathe in.
- Do not overbreathe.
- Breathe in for a count of three—pause—then exhale for a count of three.
- With each exhale, make sure you relax.
- Focus on the breath; keep that at the top of your mind.

Soon, your pain should start to subside. You may even forget about the pain as you breathe. If you start to feel lightheaded, stop and breathe normally.

Do this a couple times a day whether you are in pain or not. There are many health benefits to this diaphragmatic breathing. I recommend a "diaphragmatic breathing for pain relief" search on YouTube so you can better see how it should be done.

# Chapter Thirteen
# Cancer Blessings

**Blog Post: June 23, 2013**

It's 4:05 a.m., and I've been awake since 2:15. Just when I think three consecutive days of sleep have got me caught up, the overwhelming drowsiness hits me upside the head again. Usually, it happens when I'm ready to do something like write in my journal. Regardless, I sit here, green tea in hand, chemo cat by my side, my man snoring heavily in the next room, and I'm determined to get some thoughts out on virtual paper. Strange as it seems, this is my moment of serenity.

I've had a lot of rough moments this week. I've been too weak to do anything but saunter back and forth from bed to bathroom to kitchen. The roller coaster of emotions that go hand in hand is exhausting...DOWN, the self-pity...UP, the eager hopefulness...DOWN, the longing for the end that seems so far away. Obviously, my emotions are closely tied to my physical state. Try as I might, it is a challenge to think of blessings when your body is continually being raped by poison. Yet blessings keep popping up all around me like little dandelions, all bright and cheery yellow. I told myself I was going to make a list of cancer blessings to help remind me of all the good when I'm feeling low. Now is as good a time as any to get that list started.

Mind you, these are NOT in order of importance, just some extemporaneous thoughts bursting out of my skull as I sit here sipping green tea.

**Time to Think**. Yes, this is the biggie. I've been forced to a screeching halt. Even though this gal's overanalytical, high-speed brain runs 24/7, chemo has tamped down my ability to think quickly (chemo brain is the technical term), which makes my thoughts more methodical, deliberate, and not always accurate. At times, my thinking is less than positive, but given the circumstances, it's hard not to go down that road. I'm working on improving my positive thinking each day.

**Simple Pleasures**. Sipping green tea, my cat's purr, my lover's kiss, the soft creaky, croaky tree frog serenade outside my window, the smell of fresh cut mango, a note from a dear friend, a hug from my child, a cool breeze, savory dark chocolate, a soft rain tapping on the roof, a hearty breakfast of bacon and eggs, the ocean waves on my toes, a morning dove's repetitive coo, a cool glass of white wine (that I so dearly miss!), the humid air softly coating my skin, the vibrant colors in my healing garden ... the list seems endless.

**Love**. Ah, love ... another biggie. Dare I say cancer has shown me love? I believe it has. Several months ago, a former co-worker from Minneapolis committed suicide. I vividly recall reading the online condolences and thinking out loud, "Did she know she was this loved!?" Personally, I don't believe she did. Now that I'm in my little cancer predicament, I personally get to witness and feel such an outpouring of love from so many people. Some expected and some unexpected, but all genuinely gracious. I admit, it is a big, heady rush. My mind has been blown many a time by people's generosity, support, and their sheer desire for me to fight this demon head-on. I feel loved, but more so, I feel tremendously humbled that I am surrounded by people who love me. Outside of my inner circle, I never thought little ol' me could have any kind of impact on another person's life, but based on the love I'm receiving from so many friends, I clearly have. Don't take this wrong, but if I were to die today, I'd die knowing that I was loved. And that is the greatest gift of all.

**Prioritizing**. I believe any life-altering event is how most people come around to prioritizing what is important in life. Losing both parents, the challenges of raising a child with Asperger's & ADHD, a failed marriage that led to financial hardship, jobs that I've poured my creative heart into have all taught me an important lesson. I needed to lose to gain. It's true what "they" say: every loss has brought me something better. What I now believe is important has changed drastically from what I used to believe a few years ago. Sure, the *standards* are unchanged, like my unconditional love for Greg & my kids, their well-being—those have always been the most important. But I no longer yearn for those material things that I once thought would bring me happiness. I yearn for experiences. I yearn to embrace life full-on with reckless abandon, not sure if that is even possible, but I'm gonna give it a shot!

**Spirituality**. This goes hand in hand with love. There is a strong spiritual energy that comes from the outpouring of love that I have received. It is a HUGE blessing that I like to call Spirit Fuel. That Spirit Fuel has lifted me up when I've needed it the most. When I'm at my lowest physically and don't feel I can continue, I magically get a shot of that Spirit Fuel from someone, and my faith and belief in fighting through cancer is renewed. And if I could get all "Long Island Medium" on ya for a moment, I do feel the spiritual presence of my deceased father, mother, and grandmother, as well as my dear friend Judi, who passed from colorectal cancer at age forty-seven. I sense them surrounding me, infusing me with a loving energy to help me through this process—yet another blessing.

**Reflection**. You may think this is the same as "Time to Think," but you'd be wrong. Reflection, for me, is a spiritual retrospective. Reflecting on my past has allowed me to bring my future into focus. It has humbled me. It has shown me regret. It has inspired me. And it has made me proud of what I've done.

It's now 6:20 a.m. I hear the birds calling me to the back porch, saying, "Come and enjoy a coffee and croissant with us"…another blessing I shall partake in.

Being able to embrace your cancer blessings goes back to the mindset you carry. The many shifts I experienced during this time period offered me the ability to see the glass as half full. When cancer entered my life, that outlook became challenging.

I feel my inability to think on my feet and physically being slowed down to a pace that was unfamiliar to me assisted me in looking at the positives that I was receiving during this time.

In addition to finding my own positives, I discovered the biggest of them all—the outpouring of love, concern, well wishes, and positive vibes being sent my way. This wave of love catapulted my outlook to an even higher level. If you've never experienced being showered with unconditional care and love, then you cannot comprehend the magnitude of this gift. It can be as simple as a call, note, email, or card that lets the person know they are not alone and that they have a team of people cheering them on.

It has been a decade since my diagnosis. As I look back, I have come to believe that my cancer was truly a gift. A gift in the form of a huge lesson that redirected my life path and moved me closer to my purpose.

I carried a deep gut feeling that I needed to exit the television industry. From the time I entered management, my internal spidey sense had told me it was a bad idea, that it would eat me up, literally. And, of course, I thoroughly ignored that instinctual feeling.

During these twenty years, I internalized so much. I repressed so much anger for the many wrongdoings that were done to me, all the times my ideas and opinions were ignored or criticized, the employees who believed they could do my job better, and all the co-workers who stabbed me in the back and played nice–nice to my face. In reality, my laundry list of corporate wrongdoings committed against me was there to wake me up. To show me where I needed to speak up, call out, or walk out.

I learned through attrition that I needed to embrace my masculine side. Well, I embraced my masculine to the complete detriment of my feminine side. We carry both masculine and feminine qualities that have absolutely nothing to do with gender. Again, it's a yin-yang type of situation: you need both to be balanced. To this day, I am still working on regaining my feminine aspects. My husband lovingly calls my masculine me "corporate bitch," and he's actually spot on. So, these past few years, I have focused my energies on anchoring in my feminine qualities.

### *Prayer to Realize the Gift of Cancer*

*Dear God,*

*I am open to receiving what You wish me to learn on this cancer journey.*

*Please help me to see the gift in my suffering.*

*Open my eyes to the pain I have been needlessly taking on in my life.*

*Show me how to see the good amidst the bad*

*so that I may understand the lesson*

*my dis-ease is teaching me.*

*Creator, guide me so that I may have faith in this process.*

*I now realize that everything is designed*

*to assist us in our soul's growth.*

*Take me in Your arms so that I may navigate this*

*challenge with the highest grace and ease.*

*I am Your child, surrendering to the outcome that has yet to be revealed.*

Chapter Fourteen
# Chemo's
# Dirty Little Secrets:
# Part Two

**Blog Post: July 1, 2013**

The good, the bad, and the ugly.

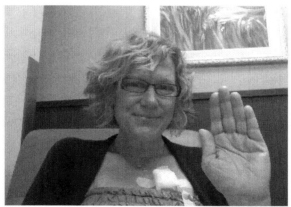
*Cycle # 5 of 12 on July 1, 2013*

Today, I sit at chemotherapy number 5. Number 4 kicked my ass. I went into the clinic during week 2 of cycle 4 and got pumped full of IV fluids. Amazingly, it really helped! I was able to get out of bed, even work half days all week!

There are so many things in your body that just don't function normally when you're going through chemo for colon cancer. I would imagine there are similarities with chemo treatments for other cancers as well. As I venture into cycle 5, I can't help but think about the good, bad, and the ugly of chemo treatments.

I am not going to start with the good. I want to end this blog on a high note. So, I'll start with the bad...

The bad is not being able to do what I've always done. I don't want to sound like a singles ad here, but I really miss walks on the beach. I'm usually too tired to take that long walk, and on top of it, I'm fearful of picking up some crazy bacteria. I'm going to have to take the risk because I just love the ocean; it's so calming. The bad is also having my friends feel sorry for me. I really hate that! Please don't shed any tears for me. As an empathetic person, I totally get it. But when it comes to me, I hate it. I don't want anyone feeling sorry for me. Why? I don't know; I just know I don't like it. What I do like and love is the supportive cards, letters, and comments I get on social media! Those are so full of positive energy and encouragement, it's great Spirit Fuel! The bad is also not being able to eat or touch anything cold. I can't tell you how much I have been craving ice cream or a big ol' milkshake! But there is no way I can eat any of that because it would feel like I was swallowing razor blades. Yep, another joy one experiences on the 5FU chemo drug.

Sadly, many of the foods I love don't love me during cancer treatment. Salads, fruits, veggies, and any other high-fiber foods wreak havoc on my system; I have to eat in moderation. Carbs seem to agree with me, which is something I didn't eat much of before. And NO sushi or ahi tuna—huge frownie face on that—too much of a bacteria risk. Go figure! Oh, and thanks to the aforementioned carbs and the steroids they add to the chemo mix, the pounds stay on ... no benefit of losing weight here. Oh, and the dreaded Chemo Brain. I've left the stove on for a few hours at a time lately. Hopefully, I don't end up burning down the house. Forming thoughts, writing, and typing is extremely difficult the first week of chemo.

The ugly is *really* ugly. Warning: if you're squeamish, then you better skip this paragraph. It's all part of the ungodly side effects of chemotherapy. For instance, losing control of one's bowels while at the Starbucks drive-thru...now, *that* is ugly. Week one, I'm bound up tighter than an Egyptian mummy. Week two, watch out...I can never be too far from a bathroom. God forbid I feel gassy, as letting one rip is **never** a good idea, as you never know what will come out with the gas! Then there are the muscle cramps and neuropathy. Some days, I feel pins and needles in my feet like they've fallen asleep. One day, my fingers started curling up and cramping; all the while, I couldn't feel them. I couldn't uncurl my fingers on my own, I needed to take one clenched-up hand to straighten my fingers out. It's terribly frightening to experience something like that, as you don't know if it's temporary or permanent!

And the good. Amazingly, there is a lot of good that can come out of the cesspool of cancer treatment. Last week Nurse Cathy was admiring my lotus tattoo as she was feeding me IV fluids. She asked if I was a practicing Buddhist. I said, "No, but I subscribe to many of their beliefs." She then told me about the Clearwater Zen Center, which she attends. The focus at the center is meditation. According to the Zen Center, the Japanese word "Zen" is derived from the Sanskrit term *dhyana*, which refers to non-dualistic, meditative absorption. Zazen, or silent Zen meditation, is the essential practice of Zen. By helping to free the mind of all thoughts and images, this practice allows our innate wisdom and compassion—our own "buddha-nature"—to come up to consciousness so that we can awaken to it and actually live the wholeness and perfection that is our birthright. Wednesday night is for beginners. I plan to attend and start getting into a regular routine of mediation. If it wasn't for Nurse Cathy, I would have been too inhibited to ever try it out! Today, I was with Nurse Theresa, who was getting me set up with my chemo IV. She asked about Noah, who was with me last time. We started talking about Asperger's and how it is hard to get him to really "get" what Mom is going through. Then she began to tell me about a boy in her Boy Scouts troop that she believes has Asperger's.

Theresa has a minor in psychology, so she knows her stuff. Turns out this troop meets just down the road from me. I've considered getting Noah into this for a while but avoided it due to his Asperger's. Well, no more! Nurse Theresa is sending me home with info and I'm getting my boy signed up as soon as I can! I can't say enough about the Walgreens Speciality Care Clinic I go to for treatment. The nurses are amazing! They are all so loving and caring; that in itself is a big part of the good! Oh, and I found out last weekend (*World War Z* spoiler alert) that zombies hate people infected with disease, so for now, I'm safe from the Zombie Apocalypse!

I want to also say thank you all for following me on this journey. Please share this blog with anyone you wish, especially anyone going through treatment and their loved ones. My hope is that by unabashedly sharing my experience it will in turn help others as they make their journey through the dark forest of Cancer and come out unscathed and healthy on the other side!

❁ ❁ ❁ ❁ ❁

## Blog Post: July 26, 2013

The bathroom chronicles, otherwise known as TMI.

Here I sit at 10:30 p.m. ....WIDE awake! I can't blame anyone; this is unintentionally self-inflicted. I drank green tea at 7 p.m., only to find out that, yes, Virginia, there is caffeine in Green Tea. DOH! Plus, my not-so-friendly bowels are in an uproar. I was supposed to be on a liquid diet for the past two days, and in a moment, I'll explain why.

Let's see, day one of the liquid diet, I made it a whole six hours before I caved and ate half a baguette loaf with butter. You would think I'd be bound up to Timbuktu after that! A couple hours later, I ate a banana and a DELICIOUS Publix brownie, the best brownie on the planet! Then, for dinner, two lovely chicken thighs. I breezed through that day and didn't have a problem until today.

Today, I went to lunch with my oldest son, Alex, who is visiting from New Mexico, along with his girlfriend, Katie, who lives in St. Louis. They asked me to lunch, and I can't pass up time with my boy and his girl! So we went to Frenchy's on Clearwater Beach. I adore Frenchy's She-crab soup, it's the BEST. Then I had chicken salad with fruit for my main course. Halfway through lunch, Alex asked why I wasn't on my liquid diet. I said I did fine for the past twenty-four hours; I think I'm OK now. Well, about an hour later, I could tell I was back on the highway to stomach hell. To top it off, Greg took me and Katie to dinner tonight at a Greek Restaurant. Again, I tried to eat blandish food, so I ordered Pastitsio that came with fresh green beans. Now, here I am at 10:30 p.m.—wide awake and running to the bathroom every fifteen minutes.

Once you get farther into your chemo treatments,

the more likely it is that your chemo weeks will get worse. At least, this is my experience with the cocktail I received for my colon cancer. I have to state that every person responds differently, every cocktail has different side effects, and every cancer and cancer treatment is different. AND I am not a doctor, nor am I giving you medical advice, you get yourself someone else for that!

I posted all my experiences on my blog, no matter how horrific, because I felt it was important for people to have some ideas on what to expect, to feel it was normal for them to experience these things because others have, and to give friends and caregivers a dose of the cancer patient's reality. If you're assisting a cancer patient who undershares, then you may want to have some idea of what they might be experiencing in silence so you can hold space for them.

In my opinion, chemotherapy is poison. A body receiving chemotherapy is working overtime to filter out and compensate for the toxic sludge that the oncologist is plugging into your veins every week or every other week. During the days/weeks you don't receive chemo, your body is going into healing mode, fighting desperately to course-correct.

I have one more chapter of these "ugly truths." This is not to create fear or dissuade you from your chemotherapy. I feel being forthcoming is the best way for everyone to get an honest depiction of what may or may not happen during chemo. Again, everybody is different. You need to dig deep and feel into what your soul is calling you to do.

### *Prayer to Embody Grace*

*Creator,*
*Show me poise in the everyday struggles.*
*Lead me through the darkness*
*and surround me in Your Light.*
*I surrender my awareness*
*so that I may witness Your miracles in motion,*
*no matter how big or how small.*
*I summon Your army of angels to surround me:*
*during my self-pity so I may embrace courage;*
*in my grief so that I may understand my true happiness;*
*while my body is swollen with pain so that I can heal;*
*during times of uncontrollable anger so that I may know peace.*
*Teach me the wisdom of Your grace so that I may one day realize the purpose of my pain.*
*It is done,*
*It is done,*
*It is done.*
*Thank You.*

## Chapter Fifteen
# Chemo Cat:
# The MiraclePurr

**Blog Post: July 6, 2013**

It's 5:15 a.m. I'm only awake because I slept most of the day yesterday. I'm sitting here, drinking my favorite zen green tea, and totally at a loss on what I should write about. Usually, I know well in advance what my subject matter will be as it is something that sits and churns in my head for a few days. Today, I got bupkis. I'm still weak from the chemo treatment. My stomach is less than cooperative. My nausea continually flairs up unless I take some antinausea meds, which knock me on my ass. It's a vicious circle of nothingness. Times like this, it's hard to keep positive because the reality is there is nothing I find too positive or eventful right now. I am merely in function mode. Sitting here on my ass, letting chemo kick my butt. Just take today and get it over with and move on to the next day and get it over with until I'm done with the damn treatment. The hard, cold truth: chemo reality bites.

Then, when I least expect it, this little fur ball

comes along and jumps on my chair…Cat Mulder. As I write this, it's like he's hearing my intuitive thoughts and makes certain his presence is known…per usual.

Mulder has become my silent nursemaid. On

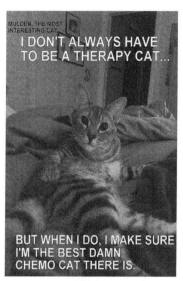

Mondays, when I come home from treatment, he is right next to me in bed, checking out my portable chemo pump and making sure I'm okay. When I get my chemo pump removed, he's back to crawling all over me, especially with his after-shower ritual where he must climb on my toweled back and balance on my shoulders like a circus cat. This is not something that can go ignored because he will pace the bathroom countertop, reaching, meowing, and waiting for me to let him on my shoulders. Odd, I know; however, I find it very amusing.

Then, on days when I'm feeling a little less wiped out, he's ready to play fetch with me. He's more of a cat-dog than a cat-cat.

Greg nicknamed him "Mulder the chemo cat." We all know about therapy dogs. So, I got to wonder if there is such a thing as therapy cats? I did a quick

Internet search and was impressed at the number of feline friends that come to the aid of humans who are dealing with difficult circumstances.

One woman's cat helped her through breast cancer. A news channel did a story on a hospital that brought 3,000 cats to a young girl undergoing cancer treatment. Personally, I was impressed to find this story about a young Asperger's girl who trained her cat to be a therapy cat, and she wishes to train more cats to help others with Asperger's. And who can resist Grumpy Cat—all that cute grumpiness is great therapy!

So, in the end, thanks to Mulder, MY therapy cat, I did have something worth writing about today!

After I lost my greyhounds, I wasn't wanting any more pets. But for years after my last cat, The Edge, passed away at eighteen, I always told my family, "My cat is going to find me." I knew there was another cat waiting to enter my life when the time was right.

After my daughter, then nineteen, moved out of the house, some boy who was trying to win her affection gave her a five-week-old kitten. My daughter would work all day, hang out with friends all night, come home, sleep, and repeat. I was watching this poor little kitten being raised as a feral cat. It broke my heart he was alone for fifteen hours a day.

First, I purchased a cat carrier and told Hannah I would cat-sit for her during the week so this cute little baby wouldn't be alone. After a couple weeks of back and forth, Greg begrudgingly said, "Just keep the cat." I was thrilled. Hannah was good with it, too, as she realized the same thing we did, that this baby needed a lot more attention than he was getting at her place.

Mulder recently turned twelve years old. This cat has taken over my whole heart. He is my soul-pet, the animal version of a soulmate. I have had many pets in my life, all of them have very special places in my heart, but this cat steals the show. His intuitive ability, the way he communicates with me without words, and his sassy, ass-cat persona, mixed with deep affection, makes him an amazing fur baby for me.

I don't necessarily recommend getting a pet when you're gearing up to go through treatment unless you have a live-in family member who is willing to take full-time responsibility for the pet *and* the patient. I could see that quickly becoming an overwhelming task for the caregiver. However, if you have a furry friend already in your home, you may be surprised at how quickly they step up to the responsibility of "therapy pet." We all know how sensitive animals are to the energy around them, so it is no surprise when a family pet senses that their human is in distress. This may be a great time to offer bed privileges to your fur baby so he/she can snuggle up next to you and offer you healing before, during, and after your treatments.

### *Blessing for Our Pets*

*Dear God,*
*Watch over our fur babies*
*as they tend to our healing.*
*Give them the added strength*
*needed during their time of service.*
*Release the pain they take from us*
*into Your energetic field*
*so that no harm comes to them.*
*I send my deepest gratitude to my pet*
*for their nurturing energy.*
*I surround my pet with my unwavering love.*
*I thank my pet for being at my side*
*so that I am not alone in my journey.*
*I am thankful.*
*I am grateful.*
*I am blessed.*

## Chapter Sixteen
# My Top 10 List.
# Half Full or Half Empty?

**Blog Post: July 16, 2013**

Day 2 of cycle 6, and I feel totally annihilated. I've been up since 4 a.m. The sleeping pills are trying to drag me back to sleep, and the steroids in my chemo are saying WAKE UP!

I lay in bed for a good hour and a half…playing on social media and thinking about all sorts of things. Mainly after viewing other people's fun, I start thinking of all the things I'm going to look forward to AFTER this damn treatment is over.

**1. Sleep!** A given. I can't say I was great at it before, but now, when I need it most, I can't get it. i.e. steroid/chemo week. And then, in the second week, out of the blue, I'll get these overwhelming feelings of sleep, like I've just walked through the Wicked Witch's poppy field.

**2. Travel.** Leaving on a plane is a no-no when your immune system is wiped out from chemo—

can't say I disagree...last place I want to be now is in a flying tin can with everyone's germs being bandied about at 30,000 feet! More so, the cruise ships I adore traveling on. They are an international hub for germs from around the world!

**3. Ice cream, smoothies, frozen yogurt, frappuccinos, Slurpees, etc.** One of my chemo drugs, fittingly called 5-FU, has a nasty side effect of not being able to drink or eat anything cold. If you do, it feels like you're swallowing razor blades. Touching it is like having thousands of needles drilled into your hands. Folks, it's been a long, hot Florida summer, and I am kinda cranky without my cool, refreshing treats!

**4. Relaxing Libations,** Zero, zip, Nada...no alcohol allowed. It is a toxic mixture when paired with chemo drugs. A very dangerous risk. Truly, the lack of libations hasn't bothered me until now...now that I see all those *cold*, refreshing beach cocktail photos that people are sipping on and posting on social media.

**5. Working Out.** Never thought I'd say that I miss working out, but I do. Last summer, through the time I was diagnosed on March 19, I was hitting the gym 5 or 6 times a week. I was obsessed but in a good way. It was great mentally, kicking that serotonin into high gear.

Physically, I liked the energy and strength I felt after my workout that kept me energized all day. Before that, I was jogging until my knee surgery in 2011 and walking daily. If I didn't do all this, how could I eat and post all those fabulous foods in my photos—I gotta offset those calories with exercise!

**6. The Beach.** There is a reason I won't leave Florida, and that is the beach! I adore the salt water and all its magnificent creatures! I love sitting in my beach chair, half in and half out of the growing tide. I love my big yellow beach umbrella. But along with all those people, there is also nastiness that can get in the water, causing abnormally high bacteria counts at certain beaches. THAT's a big risk. I have been on only one beach walk since chemo started, kept my shoes on, which sucks for this No Shoes Nation Gal. That makes me sad. Sad to keep my shoes on and sad that I just don't have much energy to do it more.

**7. Salads or Sushi.** Another anomaly for some of you, I'm sure, but I miss eating salad. In the summer, I LOVE lots of salad. At least one meal-type salad a day. Unfortunately, the damn chemo drugs jack with my system so much that it's difficult to tolerate. I have to pick and choose the days of my cycle when I think I can eat salad without suffering the repercussions. The sushi and ahi tuna are obvious ones, just can't risk any of that bad bacteria comingling with my compromised immune system. Lately, all I seem to tolerate are carbs, something I would rarely indulge in prior to chemo.

**8. Going Out & Socializing.** Just like being on a plane, going to a Rays game, a concert, a buffet, or a night club or festival are all BIG risks that frankly are not worth taking. If I get sick, that pushes my chemo treatments back, and I plan to be done with this by November!! The biggest disadvantage is not being able to go to my son's school when school starts this year. Being around children is the biggest risk, as we all know how they love to be conduits for germs! Noah is told to wash his hands and use antibacterial lotion constantly. When we go out to eat, we go off hours, like the middle of the afternoon between the lunch and dinner rush. We have also been getting more takeout if we aren't in the mood for cooking. Same goes for movies. We go a few weeks after the show has been released and try to pick off-hours. All the while making sure to sanitize, sanitize, sanitize!

**9. Hair.** I still have a decent amount of hair to date. I've been able to conceal the super thin patches with my curls. I never thought I'd say this, but this is one time I'm happy that I started off with an uber-thick head of curls. Although I still have my Raquel Welch sassy short wig on standby for when it gets TOO thin. I do look forward to growing it out again! I miss my ponytail and long Keratin-infused locks!

**10. Work.** Though admittedly, this is generally far down on my list, I do miss work. I feel like the boy in the bubble, isolated from society. I miss the creative challenges and the people. Mind you, I'm not in a rush to get back. It is worthless for me to be there and try to battle cancer at the same time. I get that I must focus on myself and my health right now!

I read this post now and I feel like it is a bunch of whiney, half-empty blah blah. I was clearly pandering to my audience, "look at all I can't do, feel sorry for me." And looking at this now, none of it is worth writing home about.

Sure, I still love to go out to eat occasionally, and the beach is great, but all I see here is a half-empty list of superficial stuff.

And when I look deeper, way underneath all I wrote, I see a woman who is not conscious of how she is living her life day to day. And I am the first to admit I wasn't. I had limited time to live because I worked ALL the time, so I just fell in line with what everyone around me was doing, eating, and drinking. I don't beat myself up for that; I actually enjoy witnessing it now. I feel so happy for that version of me, that she was able to get to where I am now.

I was curious how my list would look today, ten years later. Let's see, instead of a "what I am looking forward to after chemo" list like the one above, I'll make a what I look forward to doing in my life now (in no specific order).

**1. Snuggles, Hugs, Kisses**. Showing affection is something I no longer hold back on. I hug all my friends or new acquaintances. I snuggle my grandbabies tight. I shower my sweetie with kisses. We gain nothing and receive everything by sharing our affection.

**2. Creating**. Be it writing, painting, photography, playing music, gardening, or making something with Greg for the house, it all brings me such great joy.

**3. Nature.** Woods, beach, mountains, desert— it is all magnificent. I go stir-crazy when I am indoors too long. Nature is where I connect with spirit, where I quiet my mind and connect. Nature is where my heart is happiest.

**4. Helping Others.** I love assisting people in their awakening process and inner healing. I love sharing messages from Spirit, dragons, and angels with clients. I love when I can offer a nugget of wisdom to someone who feels stuck. I love when I can show someone the beauty I see in them. I love it when I can smile at a stranger who seems down and they smile back.

**5. Travel.** Still on my list, but what we enjoy on vacations has evolved. We love immersing ourselves in the authenticity of a place. Seeing what the people there do, what they eat, and how they live. We love exploring the local landscape of a place.

**6. Hiking and Biking.** These are done exclusively out in nature, so they are perfect. I love to move; I love to push the energy through me. I can't sit still, so these are both great ways to wear me now and allow me to enjoy the outdoors.

**7. Raising Butterflies.** It is so simple to do and so very miraculous to witness. The monarch butterfly population is suffering due to the increased use of pesticides. So every time I can raise a little caterpillar to a butterfly and set it free, my heart is so happy. And it is even happier to witness the butterflies returning to my garden and laying eggs so the cycle can continue again.

**8. A Great Meal.** For the most part, we don't eat out a lot these days. And I like to keep my body in a state of ketosis as much as I can. So when we do eat out, it needs to be great food. I will always be a foodie and have an impeccable taste for fine cuisine. I can't help it, it is one of the great joys of living in the human suit.

**9. My Cat.** Mulder, my constant companion. Greg goes away for four to five days at a time for work, and Mulder is my buddy. He was instrumental in my healing journey and continues to be. I love him like crazy.

**10. Meditation.** I love my walking meditation. It is my happy place, outdoors. It brings me peace and connects me to Spirit.

### *High Heart Meditation for Gratitude*

Begin by slowing the breath, in and out through the nose. Get comfortable. Read this meditation—putting focus on the feelings that come up when you speak these words. If you feel any emotions coming up, let them move through you. Feel them. Do not push them back down.

Move your awareness from the top of your crown (head) down to the center of your chest, your high heart.

Say the following words out loud, softly.

*My heart is an open vessel of pure Source Love. As I breathe, I drink in pure white Source Light into my high heart.*

*Breathe in and out for three counts.*

*I am grateful that eyes can see so that I may course-correct.*

*I am grateful that I can taste the sweet victory of recovery.*

*I am grateful that I can smell the pureness of grace.*

*I am grateful that my ears can hear the harmony in my positive outlook.*

*I am grateful my body can feel the dis-ease releasing.*

*I am grateful for my loving heart showing me the way.*

*Breathe in and out for three counts.*

*My dis-ease is a pathway leading me to my soul's purpose.*

*I am grateful for the lessons of my cancer journey.*

Chapter Seventeen
# And Just Like That...

**Blog Post: July 22, 2013**

I've been dealing with a specific inner struggle for a few weeks now. And even though I know it's in my best interest to just *LET IT GO*... my pit bull tendency is to latch my jaw around something and hold on tight. Once that happens, it's hard for me to release.

My issue is with what I like to call "cancer abandonment." As I write this, I'm starting to feel a bit self-centered, like everyone should pay attention to ME, and all the focus should be on ME. That is not what I'm going for here, truly! I'm talking about friends and loved ones who I believed had my back no matter what and, in some cases, all-out proclaimed that they were there for me NO MATTER WHAT. And just like that...crickets. And FYI, chances are pretty good that if you're reading this blog post, you're not one of these abandoners.

Okay, Okay, I admit that going through cancer treatment can make a person pretty needy and self-absorbed, however, isn't that the point of all this?

FOCUS on yourself, with the obvious goal of becoming cancer-free by the end of treatment? If I learned one thing from those who have preceded me on this journey, it's "No matter what, ask for help when you need it." I'm getting to the point where I need help, and I have very few folks in close proximity that I can ask. And yes, I realize that some people may have their own hang-ups with cancer, or perhaps they suffered the loss of a loved one to cancer, and now they don't have the capacity to deal with mine. To that, I'd like to add the caveat: next time, don't overpromise and underdeliver because many of us take those proclamations to heart. Like ME!

Then I jump on over to the career side of life, where there are all these wonderful little "rules" that are put in place by employers advising everyone at my level and above NOT to inquire about an employee's health or show concern for their "condition" when an employee is out on FMLA or short-term disability. This one chaps my ass because, as a manager, I truly CARE about those who are on my team, and if they were to go through an illness, I would want to show my support and concern. As you can guess, this "rule" applies to me and my current situation. God forbid corporations blur the lines and find a more "human" approach to an employee's illness. It is time to come to terms with all of it, mourn the loss of those who are not capable of keeping up, and move on. I know that it is for my own good.

Conversely, I'd be remiss if I didn't declare my absolute delight for those who lurk in the background and appear as earth angels when I need it most. Like my unassuming neighbor who is a talented BBQ pit master and shows up at my door unannounced with a heaping plate full of BBQ chicken! Or another neighbor who sees my socially challenged son riding his bike up and down the street, clearly bored that he's stuck at home this summer with his lackluster chemo mom. What does she do? Invite him to go swimming in their pool with her kids. A simple yet incredibly welcome gesture! Or sweet Erin, who offers to help me manage my rapidly decreasing hair and brings me magical banana bread to lift my spirits! And my wonderful son, Alex, who traveled across the US from New Mexico to show his support for his Ma. I am grateful and blessed to have this unforeseen help show up when I least expect it.

As I struggled to make peace with all of it, I found an excellent article on the Huffington Post website, "The Things I Wish I Were Told When I Was Diagnosed With Cancer." This article really cut to the quick, hitting on ALL the things I wish I was told! I believe it is also a great read for those who have a friend or loved one undergoing cancer treatment. Thank you, Jeff Tomczek, for this great article! I encourage you all to search it out online!

Looking back on this I can see this post was a cry for help as well as a public pity party. Geez! Here is an excellent example from *The Four Agreements*: don't take things personally!

I felt this post would serve as a perfect example of "do as I say, not as I do." I now see that I was angry. Perhaps it was more of that repressed anger I needed to release?

I no longer hold resentment or anger for those who abandoned me during my treatment. Most have naturally fallen out of my life, but on the off chance they read this book, this prayer is for you. It is called Ho'oponopono.

> I am sorry.
> Forgive me.
> Thank you.
> I love you.

Ho'oponopono is a very powerful ancient Hawaiian healing prayer. It releases memories that are experienced as problems. The practice of forgiveness is an important part of this healing. For me, it is important that I turn the resentment into forgiveness.

I have come to see this existence as one giant multi-act theatrical production being played out. And the characters that play the antagonist in your life are likely doing you the biggest favors. In the end, it always works out the way it is supposed to. The outcome may not be what you want in your human existence, but it's what your soul wanted or agreed to experience when you came here. This way of thinking may be a stretch for you, I understand; it would have been for me ten years ago, too. But this is how our major events cut us to our core. I believe they are designed to shake us awake to the true nature of our existence on this planet.

### *A Prayer to Release*
### *That Which No Longer Serves*

*Dear God,*

*Guide me with grace to release that which no longer serves.*

*As I venture down this path of healing,*

*help me recognize*

*those who support my determination to*

*release my dis-ease and heal with grace.*

*Remove those from my life*

*who cannot match my grateful view.*

*I release all these burdens to the Universe,*

*trusting that I will receive unimaginable abundance*

*in many ways, shapes, and forms.*

*I release this to You, dear God.*

## Chapter Eighteen
# The Ego and Cancer

**Blog Post: July 27, 2013**

I'm not a real fan of those who are all talk and no action, yet I feel I've become one of those people. Yeah, here I go again about the hair. I have to say to all my friends out there who gave me encouragement and told me my new "do" looks great; I appreciate that, but unfortunately, I can't agree. Right now, my hair has strictly become a matter of practicality and I hate that.

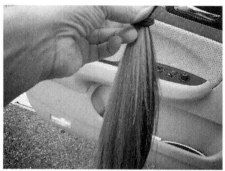

*Bye-bye, ponytail*

Any woman will attest, hair is a number one priority! After a quick Internet search, I found that the average woman spends $50,000 on her hair in her lifetime! Sounds crazy, but I'm guessing some of us will go WAY BEYOND that mark! I know personally (and fearfully) I am one who will exceed that mark. This is where Greg will likely wish I was permanently bald!

Just for fun, let's break it down:

1. Cut and style $65. Since I like long hair, I would likely do this about 4 times a year for a total of **$260**.

2. Hair products. I saw a figure on the Internet that says the average woman spends **$300** a year on products. Sadly, that sounds accurate.

3. Color. Depending on the amount of color, how many different colors, and/or number of highlights, prices can range dramatically. I would say I average about $95 a visit. Thanks to gray hair, I also visit my coiffure every 6-7 weeks, which is roughly 8.5 times a year, for a total of **$807.50**.

4. Specialty hair care. To me, this is where my Keratin Treatments come into play. Other specialty hair care could be updos, braids, conditioning treatments, etc. I get a deal on my Keratin treatments because my friend/stylist, the lovely Miss Erin, does it on the side for an average price of $250 a time, most salons charge upwards of $600 for this same treatment. For those who don't know, Keratin takes crazy curly hair like mine and makes it silky smooth and

straight—way more manageable in the Florida humidity, too! Plus, the brand Erin uses on me is free of those toxic chemicals like formaldehyde, unlike some brands. Luckily, I only get Keratin once or twice a year for a total of $**500**.

This brings the grand total to $**1,867.50** (before tips). Take that over a lifetime (roughly age 18–70), and that is 52 years of haircare which is a total of $**97,110** in my lifetime. Now, granted, I haven't been so picky about my hair in my early yearsold photos from the '80s will attest to that, and I likely won't be getting Keratin when I'm in my '60s…but damn, that is one scary figure. Ask me if I'd change anything about my hair care routine to save some coin here and there I'd say NO WAY. Hair is one of the first things people see when they meet you, aside from your face. I know what I spend on makeup is about 3% of what I spend on hair, so to me, that offsets the exorbitant price.

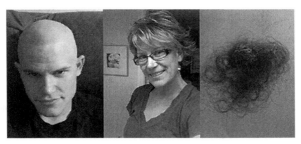

*My son shaved his head in support of*
*my ever-increasing hair loss (as seen on the right).*
*The middle pic is me in my Raquel Welch wig.*

———————————— ❧ ————————————

Yep, that was me.

Now, well…now I am *au naturale*. I maybe get a cut once or twice a year. I have completely stopped coloring my hair. I am now my natural dark brown inner mingled with lots of grey. I don't use shampoo; I clean my scalp with a Moroccan product and condition with diluted apple cider vinegar that keeps my grey hair from yellowing. And no more Keratin; I have a curly hair product so natural that I could eat it!

However, none of this is a result of my cancer journey. I apologize for burying the lead or scaring the crap out of the ladies out there.

I went back to my routine for a few years, and then 2020 happened (need I say more). I was growing weary of the constant maintenance of hair, manicures, and pedicures. Fortunately, I have never been a big makeup person, so I had that going for me. 2020 was the excuse I needed to just stop, stop all of it. So I did.

I love my grey; I actually wish I had more of it! It is quite liberating to be free of all the maintenance. Do not mistake my lack of primping and coiffing as neglect of my looks. I still like to look beautiful and dress nicely but on a level that is more fitting of my free, adventurous, nature-loving lifestyle.

A big part of my change is also due to my body no longer accepting most chemicals. The last year of coloring, I would go home to terrible itching of my scalp for days. Then, that started happening with shampoos as well.

As I moved to remove as many inorganic products as possible from my life, it was a truly natural transition.

I recently heard that hairs are like antennae that gather and channel the sun's energy and move to the frontal lobes of the brain that we use for meditation or visualization. These antennae act as conduits, bringing in subtle cosmic energy. And, apparently, it takes three years from your last cut for your antenna to form at the tip of your hair. I take this with a grain of salt as I know plenty of people with short hair or no hair who are very connected to the cosmos and are beautiful conduits for Creation.

Hair isn't the only thing that you'll be faced with altering or changing during your cancer journey.

Most days, I wouldn't want to look in the mirror. I literally had no clue who this person was looking back at me. I felt unrecognizable. I felt hollow.

My healing journey around my appearance has been lifelong. It was distorted in my youth. And cancer exacerbates that process. I will likely be working on deprogramming my issues around my appearance until the day I die. The pressure on women to look youthful is still enormous. And once women get to a certain age, they are discarded and hidden from the public eye. Media tells us this, so it must be.

It hurt me to see myself after cancer. I was mentally and physically drained of my essence. I didn't feel attractive. No matter how often Greg told me I was beautiful, I felt like my body was swapped out for an inferior model when I wasn't looking.

The year after chemo, I noticed that my skin took a big hit. I went from firm skin, toned, and tanned skin to crinkly, crepey skin. The blotchy spots eventually faded. My stamina took a good year to return. And my sex life, well, it was slow to return, and when it did, it was far tamer than it used to be.

I was growing into a deeper state of spiritual awareness, which was wonderful, but let's get real: I was also sad that I had lost my youth virtually overnight. So, I had to mourn the loss of who I once was. I have moved through most of that, but I get caught occasionally when I glance in the mirror and see this older version of me staring back. My mind, body, and soul feel so youthful now; I just need to figure out how to naturally reverse-age my appearance!

Chapter Nineteen
# Chemo's
# Dirty Little Secrets:
# Part Three

**Blog Post: August 11, 2013**

The Cat and the Shat; the painful realities of a foodie going through chemo.

Here I sit at 3 a.m....awake again. I am partially to blame, maybe like 25%. The other 75% is chemotherapy's fault. You see, I'm a big-time foodie. I love really good food. I love to critique food. I even had a food blog for a brief moment in time (chomping-at-the-bit.blogspot.com, which lasted two months... squirrel!). I most definitely LOVE to take pictures of pretty food! Last night was no exception. I took my man out for what I guess would be our anniversary, 8.12.2010. The actual day is Monday, but that is my chemo day. We're not married, so I celebrate the day I first emailed him after twenty-six years apart, the stars aligned, and our lives congealed into a spectacular jello mold of love. See, I can't even write without thinking of food. And I'm not even sure that Greg would notice if the day came and went without celebration. Me, on the other hand, I love *any* reason to go out and celebrate our love over good food.

We had dinner at Marlin Darlin', a local Key West-style dinner establishment. We hit the joint right at 4 p.m. when they opened. No, I'm not an early bird with my AARP card (yet!); it's a trick I like to use to try and keep myself out of big crowds. The fewer people I'm around and the more I hand sanitize, the better! That way, I lower the risk of catching a bug that would set my chemo back a few weeks. Anyway…I ordered Grouper Cheeks Piccata, a linguine with a lemony caper sauce and tiny grape tomatoes. The grouper was broiled perfectly. It wasn't spicy, and I thought it was something my stomach could handle. Guess what? I was wrong. So here I sit at 3 a.m., literally running to the bathroom every ten minutes like an Olympic sprinter, trying not to shit my pants! Don't laugh; it's a true fact and has happened to me a few times! It's just one of the many ugly truths that a lot of chemo patients deal with on a regular basis.

As I sit here, waiting to make another mad dash to the latrine, I can't help but imagine that this is a spell from a wicked foodie witch somewhere! She hates my love for food so much that she has placed a curse on me! Actually, the witch is a bitch, and her name is chemo! I hate these harsh realities and the army of side effects that come along with them. It's more fun to make up stories in my head about wicked witches.

I have chemo cycle number 8 on Monday. I'm dreading the horrible week ahead yet relishing the fact that I'll be done after four more cycles (that's two months), barring any unforeseen circumstances such as low blood counts or getting sick. It's far better to be on the downward slope of chemotherapy than the other side. If you're on the uphill climb, don't fret; just take it day by day. It really is the ONLY thing you can do. Try to occupy that chemo brain with something. Books are hard to read right now. Even watching TV for more than an hour is difficult. Personally, I occupy myself with writing, which is very cathartic, or I just sit on my back porch, watching the birds at the feeder, gazing at my healing garden, or enjoying an afternoon rain shower. Chemo makes you slow waaaaaay down, so do just that. Relax and relish the slow pace of life right now.

❦ ❦ ❦ ❦ ❦

## Blog Post: August 23, 2013

Here I am, again, in this vicious circle… off to bed at 8 p.m. and wide awake by 10:30 p.m. I used to make it a good five hours. The last two nights, it's been two hours max! Not cool.

With chemo, it's hard to track down the "source" of ailments. I stopped drinking caffeine late afternoon, but my God, how much caffeine can be in green tea? The post-chemo meds last week were changed up, so

I'm not taking as many steroids, but perhaps there is a lingering effect? I've had energy for the past two days and organized a couple closets in the house... one would think that would wear me out, and it did, but not enough to sleep a whole night. Nope. I have no clue what the culprit is. So, here I sit.

The frustrating thing about chemo is not knowing how you'll react on any given day or week. Last round was frightful! I spent most of the two weeks in the bathroom. Knowing I didn't want to endure that again, I changed up my diet for this cycle and omitted any salads, fruits, veggies, and coffee. Surprisingly, that did the trick (so far)! I hate it, though, because those are some of my summer eating favorites!

I also hate what the steroids do to my body. Suffice it to say I'm pushing a good twenty pounds heavier without eating more than I have pre-chemo, thanks to the steroids. I usually have one filling meal a day, then snack on small stuff like yogurt, granola bars, or crackers the rest of the day. But given my lack of activity, I'm certainly not burning up calories. It's mostly frustrating as I do NOT want to buy clothes that are bigger when I plan to work at shrinking and losing those LB's once chemo is over.

The good thing is I do believe the fluids I received last week when I was dehydrated have helped me have a good week this week. Last week, when I went in to have my portable pump removed, the nurse could tell I was in bad shape. She took my BP, and it was

80/50. Then she took my pulse, which was over 100. A combo that apparently dictates one is dehydrated. And yes, another lovely chemo side effect is dehydration. I can drink a gallon of water a day, but my body absorbs water differently while I'm on chemo. My body pretty much does everything different while I'm on chemo! So, although I'm drinking a lot, it's not necessarily doing what it should, so the boost of a couple liters of fluids pumped directly into my bloodstream has done WONDERS! My unsolicited advice to my chemoites: get fluids when you're run down or feeling like you're on the verge of dehydration. It should do wonders for you, too!

Thanks for following! This little blogger is off to attempt shut-eye AGAIN! Wish me luck! xo

❧ ❧ ❧ ❧ ❧

## Blog Post: September 27, 2013

As I round the corner to chemo #11 on October 7, I start pondering my recovery. I wish that the day after my last treatment that everything in my body will magically revert back to my old self (minus the cancer, of course). Unfortunately, it will be months until I'm feeling like a non-chemo-laden, positive, post-cancer gal. The nasty chemo has done a number on my body. Now, I know everyone has different reactions to chemotherapy, as different cancers call for different types of chemo drugs. What I'm sharing today is MY reactions to my chemo treatments for colon cancer and how it affects me. You or your loved one's side effects may or may not be similar.

I'll start with my **feet/hands**. One side effect that I had only one time was my feet swelling up like big ol' sausages. The left foot was worse than the right. The doc prescribed something and it went down in about three days. The BIGGER issue with my feet is numbness—which also affects my fingers. This problem has been getting worse with each treatment. So much so that on treatment number 10, the oncologist reduced my 5FU by 25%. Sorry to say, that didn't help, and the numbness is only increasing. This side effect can last months, years, or be permanent after chemo. It is one that the doctors try to monitor very closely. God forbid I lose more feeling. It's hard to be on my feet too long when they are numb, and just typing this right now is awkward as I'm continually missing keys and have a pins and needles sensation in my fingertips.

**Knees/weight/eating habits**. My knees are puffed up and look like old lady knees. Actually, my whole body is puffed up to the tune of twenty pounds, thanks to the steroids in the chemo drugs. Finding food that agrees with your digestive system during chemo is not easy. I learned the hard way (days spent chained to the toilet) that I can't eat salads, fruits, veggies, or consume too much coffee on certain days during treatment. My diet primarily consists of carbs (ugh). Easy to pack on twenty pounds with that diet!! Drinking fluids is uber-important, too! I learned that the hard way by getting dehydrated a few times. Gatorade is now a regular part of my day.

**Hair loss**. This one is the worst, in my opinion. I have always struggled with my crazy curly hair until a couple years ago when I found out about Keratin Treatments! Since then I've loved my hair, only to lose it all with chemo. Okay, I didn't lose ALL of it, but there are big patches of baldness all over my head, and my hair is very thin and wiry.

**Skin**. Your skin gets awful during chemo! I have cellulite where I never had it or imagined I'd ever have it. My skin is dry all the time. Any cuts or sores take a long, long time to heal. I constantly have raggedy cuticles. Oh, and I have this charming rash that started on my arms, has moved to my chest, and is slowly working its way onto my face. It looks like chicken pox. This may or may not go away after treatment. This was not a side effect the chemo nurses or my doctor have seen before.

**Muscles/joints**. My knees, joints, and lower back ache a lot. Those have been problem areas for me in the past, so I'm guessing chemo amplifies any aches and pains in those areas. Getting in and out of my car, which may be a little on the low side, makes me feel like an eighty-year-old.

**Fingernails**. Some people lose their fingernails during treatment, and others have their fingernails go hog-wild, growing like crazy. I got the grow-like-crazy nails. This would be great if I was allowed to get manicures and grow them long, but long nails hold germs under them, so you gotta keep them short. And manicures open you up for infections from even the most sterilized manicure tools.

**Stomach/Bowels**. This one is not for those who get queasy, so if that is you, you may want to skip this paragraph. I believe it's important to be very transparent about what can happen to a body during chemo, so here goes. As mentioned earlier, your stomach will not tolerate certain foods. You'll need to learn to gauge that on your own by trial and error. I used to have major constipation on week one of chemo. By week two, I could be living on the toilet with diarrhea. And some days, getting to the toilet in time was impossible. I'm not talking about a shart, folks. I'm talking about sneaky liquid poo that shoots out of your bunghole without ANY warning. It's times like that when I was glad to be home on short-term disability! Learning what I could eat and drink eventually helped me avoid problems, but it was a steep learning curve for a while.

**Teeth/Nose and other orifices**. During chemo, your membranes get weak and tender. Usually, the first week of chemo is the worst. I'd blown my nose and had bloody noses as a result. I'd brushed my teeth, and my gums will bleed. I've even bled like a young, virginal girl after being intimate with my lover. You just never know when it will happen. You just need to take it easy on your orifices!

**Brain**. Ah, my favorite (she says sarcastically) …chemo brain. No, it's not a cute phrase; it's an actual medical side effect of chemo. It's a lot like a slow-mo version of A.D.D. Your brain is foggy a lot. You forget the simplest things, sometimes mid-sentence. Concentration for an extended period of time is difficult. You don't react as quickly. God forbid you needed to have a debate when you have chemo brain, it just wouldn't end pretty.

**Sleep**. For many, sleep may be difficult. As if the anxiety and stress of having cancer isn't enough, the steroids they pump in you during week one may have you up at night. In the beginning, that was the case for me, so they cut me back a bit, and now, when I'm at home with the portable pump, I pretty much sleep constantly.

I hope this didn't come across as a long diatribe of complaints. My goal is to help you glean some information that may help you or your loved one have an idea of what to expect when it comes to side effects. If you ever have any problems, talk to your chemo nurse; they are amazing and so very helpful. They will likely have some tips and tricks to help you out.

I'll say it again, chemotherapy is poison. Look at it like a hero going off to war. That soldier will likely take down, kill, or attempt to take down many enemies. That soldier will also unwittingly take many civilian lives in the process. Chemo will likely kill the enemy cancer cells, but it will also affect other healthy areas of your body that you depend on.

Knowing what I know now, if I were to go back and do it all over again, I would first examine my own state of being, mentally, physically, and spiritually. I would closely examine all the things in my life that may contribute to my disease on all three of those levels. There is a reason this is called a disease: it is creating _dis-ease_ in your body.

I have come to believe over the years that our environment and the stress we carry are the biggest contributors to our dis-ease or to our well-being. Many of you will not subscribe to this statement. You may take a victim stance, but what if I was to tell you that I once believed I was a victim, too? I held the belief that I was not in control of my own life, that random, horrible things were cast upon me. I now see that my victimhood was merely a story that I told to try and justify the poor decisions that I made in my life. I would try and justify why I ate fast food: I was so busy and too important to take the time to cook healthy. I subscribed to the Western medical ideology that was designed to keep me dependent on pills rather than to show me how to heal myself. I told myself a story that others' negativity stormed over me like a hurricane, infecting me with discourse that created my disease, when in reality, I was the one fueling my own storm.

You are the best judge of what treatment you are willing to put your mind, body, and soul through. It should never be a rushed decision. It should be completely YOUR decision, not your partner's, not your children's, not your parents', it should be yours! Weigh all the information and then tap into your inner knowing. Talk to your soul. Ask God and your angels for advice. You're not alone on this journey; however, the decision of where this journey takes you is one hundred percent yours.

*Dear God,*

*Deliver me from the dis-ease in my life.*

*Give me the clarity to see that I am worthy of*

*love, of being heard, of thoughtful compassion.*

*Bring me to a place of peace so that I may see that the place in which I reside is not for my highest and best good.*

*Assist me in following through on making that best choices to serve and maintain my vessel.*

*I summon Your angels above to walk me down a path of health and well-being,*

*for my mind,*

*for my body,*

*and for my spirit.*

*I put my trust in You, dear God.*

*Thank You.*

# Chapter Twenty
# Good Amidst the Bad

**Blog Post: October 12, 2013**

The past three days, I have been taking walks (per Oncologist's orders) to try and alleviate the numbness in my feet. I have also been exercising my hands for that same reason. It's been a week, and I haven't noticed *any* difference. It's quite frustrating to feel constant numbness in my extremities. I can't begin to tell you how many times a day I trip or drop things. My hope is it won't be permanent, but that is an ugly truth I may need to come to terms with at some point.

I can also tell my blood count is still low. I still tire easily and still crave my midday nap! I have been reading on ways to get my white blood count up. I hate to go back to work with it low and get exposed to all the germs and sickness that seem to go along with an enclosed office environment. Getting sick is not something I care to deal with at this time—or anytime, really!

I don't want to be a Debbie Downer, that is not my goal, so here is some positive news to offset the negative! My digestive system has regulated itself back to where it once was and I can now eat salads and fruits again! I'm currently eating lots of protein to get my red and white blood counts up and give me energy. I'm also working on eliminating sugar and refined carbs, which is never easy. It's a process, and I'll eventually make it back to my healthier eating habits! Right now I'm just happy to have my salads back!!

The walks I'm taking at the park across the street are not only good for my body; I'm finding that they are good for my soul as well. The sweltering Florida humidity has left, and the mornings have been simply perfect! Not to mention, taking in ANY scenery that isn't my backyard is pretty nice at this point!

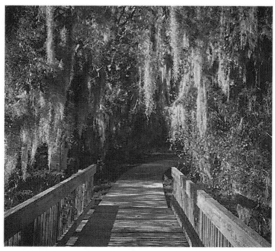

*My daily healing walk.*

I look back on this post and realize that I was being led by the healing power of nature. Nature has become an amazing tool for my healing on this journey. The practice has become *second nature* to me.

Today, I head out on the hiking trail early. I find that the morning is the best time for me to receive my musings. The meadow leading into the woods is blanketed in a thick layer of fog, it looks so etheric and magical.

I am always awestruck by nature. From the sheer force of her storms to the gentleness of her trees swaying in the wind. She can go from wreaking havoc to pure blissful serenity. She is an amazing force and she is also a welcoming mother, offering healing to anyone willing to step into her office and accept her remedies.

Since I was a little girl, the outdoors have been my happy place. I would spend hours in our backyard playing in my mother's flower garden, running in circles around the tulips with my dog, Hilda. It always felt more natural for me to be in nature.

I feel the same way now every time I walk through the forest. I dream of building a tiny, secret cabin back among the pine trees, tucking it in just right so no one can find me.

As I walk down the trail, I see the silhouettes of two does up ahead. As I keep walking, a group of five deer leap across the trail only 100 feet in front of me. The power of their being, their hooves hitting the ground, their little white tails bouncing through the brush as they scamper away from me, it is like I am witness to something as precious as the discovery of gold. My heart expands wide open with excitement. I walk the rest of the trail, gobsmacked by the power of these amazing creatures. Times like this make me feel so grateful that I can walk amongst the trees, the animals, and the wildflowers.

I love modern conveniences as much as the next person, but the more time I spend in nature, the more I see the programming and the trappings of our manmade existence. And at the time of writing this book, we are entering into the age of artificial intelligence. I try to observe this "innovation"; however, my intuitive instincts feel all knotted up at the thought of where this could lead humanity. Why would we want to create an artificial intelligence when man isn't even using the intelligence he has been given by our Creator? These robots are only as good and only as benevolent as the people making them, and I wonder, I truly wonder, how benevolent the makers of AI are.

So I released that thought into an observation. I know the only thing that I can control, that I can manipulate, and that I can ever do is focus on me. And this is where nature truly enhances my state of being.

I continue down the path, and I see a beautiful hawk feather lying in front of me. I collect all these feathers and view them as offerings, beautiful gifts from the wilderness. I always get giddy like a child on Christmas morning every time I come across a feather. They are so precious to me!

Over the years, as I spend more time hiking in the woods, I have found that this is where I can most easily connect to my inner self/higher self. I have been able to receive messages from benevolent beings and collectives who are here to assist in our planetary shift. Many refer to this as channeling. The pine trees act as antennae connecting me to the ethers as I walk among them.

Now, for those who feel a little weirded-out by the word channeling. Know that it is actually a very natural process when you are heart-centered and emanating love. Sometimes it comes on naturally, and you may not even be aware you're channeling. You may think they're just thoughts rolling through your mind when truly they are heart-centered messages coming in from the beyond.

Have you ever watched a musician who is so into his music and just rolling through a magnificent melody, so much so that he doesn't even seem like he's aware of what he's doing? To me, that is a form of channeling. Or an artist splashing paint across a canvas, so in the moment that they aren't even conscious until they stand back and view their magnificent piece of art. It's being in the flow and receiving what a higher dimensional assistance is bringing through. It's a form of channeling.

I feel there is so much that we as humans are capable of if we could just get out of our own way, if we could see the beauty and the love in everything around us. I never intended on channeling anything until I did. I was simply trusting and leaning in to a state of flow, letting my soul drink and all the beauty of my natural surroundings as I was walking in nature.

The woods is my church, the birds are my choir, the deer are the deacon, walking me down the Lord's path. And every day, my heart is open to receiving this awe-inspiring communion. When you can be in a true state of pure gratitude for every step that is in front of you, this is when you can hear the angels speak.

I wrote this chapter at the end of March 2023 and looked back at where I was ten years ago. I was days away from receiving my cancer diagnosis. Today, I am taking a six-mile hike through my church, reveling in the splendor of my beautiful pine tree cathedral. I can see God in everything, well, almost everything—I'm having a really hard time seeing God in this annoying horsefly that's been dive-bombing in my head.

Sometimes, when I'm feeling in a funk or sadness washes over me from something that is out of my control, I come out to the woods to release my angst. And one hundred percent of the time, I always leave feeling uplifted and grateful, with loving understanding in my heart. And many of those times when I have come into the words to seek an answer or ask for a sign, something miraculous is always given to me… always. Whether it's a beautiful feather from a majestic bird, or a barred owl appearing in my path, or even a family of otters scampering across the trail in front of me, these are all beautiful signs and confirmations for me. And the cool thing is, they are just for me.

Next time you're in the woods, drop into your heart space, and ask for some sort of confirmation or sign for something that you may be working through, and then just watch what happens. Did you see something you haven't seen before? Did you notice a flower that seems new to you? Did you hear something that you haven't heard when you've been out in nature before? Did you look up and happen to notice a bird that you hadn't seen on previous walks? Be open, be accepting of whatever you receive, and you will always receive as long as your eyes, ears, and heart are open.

### *Nature's Prayer*

*Dear Mother Earth,*

*My heart resides within your woodlands as I find solace among your pines.*

*I drop to my knees, feeling your soft dirt against my skin, I pray for healing.*

*The canopy of trees above looks down upon me with their blessings.*

*I hear the heavenly songs of angels with every bluebird's graceful melody.*

*Gently cradle my spirit within your clouds so that I may feel the winds of freedom.*

*Envelop me in your streams, lakes, and oceans; baptize me as your earthen child.*

*I release my soul to the expansiveness of your kingdom.*

*Thy will be done, dear Mother.*

# Chapter Twenty-One
# Cancer Lessons

**Blog Post: October 16, 2013**

The other day at breakfast, Greg asked me what I've learned from going through my cancer treatment. When cancer presented itself, my goal was to find "Zen" during my treatment, but I had yet to stop and really consider what I'd learned. Maybe it's still too early in the process, and my lesson has yet to present itself; you know, "hindsight is 20/20." I have to admit, I expected the heavens to part and some great epiphany to hit me at the end of chemotherapy. Well, that never happened. Now I feel like a dolt!

So, after the question was posed, I pondered for a while and know that I have learned some lessons during chemotherapy. None of them grand by any means, but they are lessons I've stumbled upon nonetheless and might be helpful to others who are going through cancer treatment. Here they are.

**Chemotherapy nurses are angels sent from God**. Yep, they are intuitive, wise, and immensely caring people. Honor and respect them always! And bringing them treats once in a while is a great idea, too!

**You may feel like you're dying, but you'll be treated like a rockstar**. People will shower you with gifts, bend over backward to help you out, and give you oodles of encouragement. Take it all. Feel blessed. The love from others, however it's presented to you, is given to get you through this hell on earth.

**Someone always has it worse**. I learned this from my gracious guest bloggers, Cory, Ray, Tom, Sue, Amy, and Belle. I applaud their wherewithal and courage. They have been dealt some hefty cancer cards and are embracing life in spite of cancer. They are my heroes, and I am proud to call them friends!

**Don't be stubborn; seek help!** I am fortunate enough to realize there are some issues in life too big for me to take on by myself. I am not Wonder Woman. Hence why I reached out to Immerman Angels and requested an earthly angel's assistant. My wish was granted with Lee. She too is a gift sent from God. She is open and very responsive to all my questions. She pays attention to where I'm at in the chemo process and knows the right questions to ask. She has many helpful suggestions for dealing with ailments during treatment. And she's just an all-around sweet person who I can call my angel and my friend!

**Put it in low gear and keep it there**. If you're a type A personality, like me, you'll have a hard time letting stuff go and operating at a snail's pace during chemotherapy, but it is necessary! Most times you'll be forced into submission as your body will now allow you to do anything but be bedridden. But when you get that rare feeling like you can get up and do something, just take it slow and don't overdo it. REST as much as you can!

**It's OK to melt down**. I had more than a few meltdowns over the last six months. It's daunting to find out you have a disease that can end your life. It's also a tremendous physical and mental burden to take on chemotherapy! At some point, you'll need to cleanse your heart and soul with tears so you can rid yourself of the negative thoughts and hopefully move toward the positive mindset you'll need to fight the battle of your life. Mind you, it IS a roller coaster ride ALL the way through treatment and even during the recovery stage. Just know it's OK to succumb to the anger and sadness once in a while so you can get it out of your system and move on to a better state of mind.

**Kick your caregiver(s) out of the house.** OK, not permanently, just for a few hours now and again. It is important to be cognizant of the toll chemo takes on those close to you. It took some minor meltdowns between Greg and me before we realized he needed to get out of the house so he could recharge. Watching a loved one endure cancer treatment is very stressful. So, Greg finally took in a few baseball games and some long bike rides, and we started hitting the gym again, which I think was a big help.

**Life is too important to be taken seriously.** I look back at some of the intense stuff that I've had to deal with over the past decade and wonder if I could have gotten through it in a less dramatic fashion. Some of it, probably not. Other issues that were less intense, probably so. Cancer has taught me that I need to lighten up. I tend to take some things too seriously. Am I there yet? Hell, no. I am a work in progress. All I can do is be present in each moment and try to remember there are more important things in life.

**Lighten up your load**. (This may not be for everyone.) I had a lot of time to lay around and ponder my life during chemotherapy. I thought about some of the amazing experiences I've had with Greg since we reunited. I wouldn't trade those for anything. Then I got to looking at all the "stuff" I've accumulated over the years. Stuff I now believe was purchased to fill a void in my life. Recently, I've started purging my stuff, and it feels so good. Every year, I try to unload more and more until I can get down to the bare essentials, and that is NOT easy. My new motto: clear the clutter and clear my mind! I want to lighten my load so I can put my energy (and cash flow) toward experiences. If nothing else, my goal is to die with my boots on!

**The only people you need in life are the ones who need *you* in their lives, even when you have nothing left to offer**. I was warned that some of the people you thought for sure would be there for you and be supportive through chemotherapy are sometimes the ones who are quick to abandon you in your time of need. I really couldn't fathom that idea until it happened to me. However, there is a flip side to this...there are people you never expected to step up and be uber supportive who do so in a heartbeat. I was blessed enough to be on the receiving end of that experience, and for that, I am grateful. This experience is how you find your true friends for life!

**Spread an attitude of gratitude.** I feel blessed that my stage-3 cancer was caught probably at the earliest possible moment that you can diagnose stage-3 cancer. If you recall, my doctors thought I just had some benign polyps that needed removing. Then, when one was cancerous, they thought, we'll remove that section of the colon (due to my family history, they wanted to treat it aggressively), and then I'd be done with it. THEN, when they removed lymph nodes along with the eighteen-inch section of the colon, they found cancer in two of fifteen of the lymph nodes! I am not a doctor, but to me, that seems pretty damn early to catch a stage-3 cancer. I'm placing my bets that chemo knocked out any other rogue cancer cells floating around my body! I am grateful for my primary physician, who all but walked me to the gastroenterologist's office! I'm grateful for my surgeon, my gastroenterologist, my oncologist, and all the caring nurses I met along the way. I'm grateful for family and friends who supported me. I'm grateful for my true love, who put up with more than his fair share of Linda the last six months. The list goes on and on, but you get my point. PROCLAIM your gratitude to those who helped you and anyone around you who will listen. It's a great way to manifest positive energy!

**Live life to the fullest every chance you get!** You know the saying, "Dance like no one is watching"? That is what I'm going for! You shouldn't give a shit what others think about how you live your life. Wear your freak flag proudly!

Do the things that bring you joy! I am pondering some changes in my life that I am sure will make many scratch their heads and wonder why, but I don't give a rat's ass. I believe I was given the gift of more years on this planet, and I don't want to squander them! Face it, whether you have cancer or not, everyone deserves to find their bliss! Now get off this blog and go uncover yours!

If I were to tell you that I am grateful for my cancer diagnosis, what would you think?

Well, I'm here to tell you I am grateful for my cancer diagnosis. I am also grateful for my failed marriage. I am grateful for my exit from my six-figure-a-year salary in the corporate world. I am grateful for going through the process of chemotherapy (even though I would never do it again). I am grateful for all of these things and so much more!

When I learned to release my victim mentality, I was able to stand back and objectively look at all of my perceived failures, traumas, and dramas through a lens of neutrality and receive these events as beautiful learning opportunities. Everything that I deemed as "bad" that happened to me was really a fast-track lesson for me to upgrade myself in this human existence. I now carry so much compassion for all of those whom I perceived as wrongdoers. I now take a 10,000-

foot view of them from a higher vantage point. I can clearly see their pain and trauma. I can see their distant desire for healing. I can see what we did to each other (because, honey, it takes two to tango) and that we were both operating from a place of pain and suffering. I now look back on these magnificent teachers, and I can applaud their Oscar-winning performances. And then I imagine the day when our souls all meet again, in the void of the ethers, when we are surrounded by pure love and bliss, and I will thank them for their amazing service to my soul's expansion. And we will laugh, and we will party, and we will be so grateful for all the lessons that we taught and learned from one another here on Earth.

Until that day comes, however, I will practice using a lens of neutrality in situations that arise. Observing through a place of non-judgment, and digging into the possible lesson that each situation is offering me. Again, this is one of those "easier-said-than-done" practices that will take a lifetime to perfect. I believe if you can get to a state of awareness around your thoughts, that's half the battle. I am the first to admit that I am far from perfect, but I have gotten pretty good at noticing and catching myself saying things that may be judgmental or voicing the thoughts of the ego-mind. The last thing you should do is beat yourself up for that because the pure awareness around catching yourself is a huge accomplishment!

As humans, we think we may have a grand and

magnificent purpose to fulfill during our time on the planet. But consider that perhaps we came here to become more aware of judgments and negative self-talk. Imagine if you were able to catch yourself doing those things ... now you have just assisted in exponentially raising the vibration of this planet. And that's just one example. Yes, we like to believe in the grandiose missions, but what Spirit perceives as grandiose may be as simple as bringing yourself into the awareness of your thoughts.

As time marches on, my lessons from my cancer journey continue to expand as my consciousness expands. I look back now on what I see as simple lessons for my blog post in 2013, but those simple lessons were beautiful mustard seeds that grew into the expansion that my soul is now experiencing ten years later.

My intention is to keep expanding, keep learning, and keep growing in my awareness, in my love, and in my compassion for humanity. And I'll tell you, these are not easy tasks! I am not a people person. I very much like my alone time. I enjoy sitting in quiet contemplation. And I am so happy when I am just able to move through the flow of any given day without a single item on my agenda. Then I am reminded that, "Hellooooo, you came to earth to experience all these people, places, and things!" Yes, indeed I did!

It's a fine balance to walk between a practice of ascending in consciousness versus enjoying the buffet of 3-D experiences that planet Earth has to offer us.

If I had to drill it down to the biggest lessons over these past ten years as I move farther away from my cancer diagnosis, I would have to say it is the lesson of letting go.

*Letting go of expectations.*

*Letting go of petty arguments.*

*Letting go of negative thoughts.*

*Letting go of grudges.*

*Letting go of anger.*

*Letting go of the idea of perfection.*

*Letting go of what others will think.*

*Letting go of needing to be right.*

*Letting go of fighting and arguing.*

*Letting go of watching or reading the news.*

The *letting go list* could go on for eternity. I would recommend that perhaps you make your own list and see what is worth letting go of for you.

In the end, if you can look at yourself in the mirror, directly in your eyes, and say, "Today I did the absolute best that I could," then you are doing a great job!

## Chapter Twenty-Two
# Remnants Remain

**Blog Post: November 19, 2013**

I'm into my third week back at work. It's nice to be busy again. For the most part, I forget about the cancer except when my neuropathy shoots me a painful reminder in the foot or hand. Plus, I am assuming this is related to my nervous system being ravaged, I startle so easily! If I don't catch someone out of my peripheral vision and they come up behind me unnoticed, I literally jump out of my skin!

I always dreamed of the day chemo ended when I was going through treatment. Just six months ago, I saw myself at the completion of a long journey, being happy and resuming my pre-chemo life. Little did I know the chemo cocktail that was designed to cure my cancer would also give me potential lifelong side effects. And so, my journey toward healing continues. Is it life-threatening? No. Is it life-altering? Yes. I was an active gal who is now being slowed down by more challenges. I want to believe I can overcome this obstacle as well, but when I need my guy to hook my bra strap every morning, it's a bit discouraging.

Regardless, this was the week of two significant doctor appointments. One to see a neurologist and one to get my port removed.

On Monday the neurologist spent over an hour with me, reviewing symptoms and testing my hands, feet and legs. The bad news is the extent of my neuropathy is "quite significant" (my doctor's words). The worst part starts at my toes and covers my feet to my ankles. For example, during one of the tests I couldn't tell which direction she was moving my toes. To a lesser degree, the damage extends up to my knees. It is also prominent in my fingertips. For some reason, the damage finds the nerves farthest from the brain, which are in the the feet, and then works its way up the body. I also have damage in my fingertips because when my arms are at my side, my fingers are close to reaching my knees, thus making those nerves a considerable distance from the brain as well and a good place for the nerve damage to take up residence. I asked why I wasn't seeing any improvement since my last chemo, and that is because the nerves only heal a millimeter at a time. The doctor said to measure my recovery in months, not weeks. So, four months from now, I should assess my improvement compared to today. The not-so-reassuring part was that the chemo patients she has had over the years generally saw only a 40-60 % improvement in symptoms. Sorry, but I am ready to have a 95-100% improvement...so watch out, shitty statistics, I'm gunning for ya!!

The next step is trying to find the best way to

work toward healing my nerve damage, which is a neuroconduction test and an EMG test. From what I understand (and you should look it up yourself as I am no medical specialist), the neuron-conduction test is electrodes that are hooked up to my body and electrify my nerves while measuring the results, thus learning the extent of the damage and where to focus treatment. The EMG test involves getting stabbed with needles all over the worst areas of my feet and hands, another way to narrow down the nerves that are damaged. Hmmm, getting electrocuted and stabbed…sounds like fun!

I will also be starting physical therapy and occupational therapy. The importance of PT is to make sure I learn how to work with my newly numbed feet. I could easily hurt myself, so I need to develop techniques to stay safe and not cause any permanent damage to other parts of my body by falling or twisting joints. The OT is to learn how to work within the confines of my numbness by learning techniques for everyday living, such as writing longhand and getting dressed (buttons, hooks, etc.).

My favorite doctor appointment this week was getting my port out! The procedure was interesting. I had to go under anesthesia to have the port "installed," but only had a local anesthetic to have the port removed. The worst part was the shot to numb the area; the rest I never felt. I now have one less reminder of my torturous journey. An important step forward as I work to move further away from the remnants of cancer.

As time moves on, I find that there are quite a few remnants of chemo that continue to crop up and affect my body and my life.

The most notable one as of late was my need to have cataract surgery at fifty-seven years old. I had my eye-glass prescription updated at the end of October. By the beginning of December, when I picked up my new glasses, I still had blurred vision in my right eye. I received a revised prescription and another pair of new glasses in January, and still my eye was blurry. My eye doctor took another look at my eyes and it was finally clear to her that I had cataracts in my eye. The right one was very pronounced. But once you have one eye corrected, you need to have the second one done as well in order to even out your vision.

I was beyond frustrated to know I needed surgery on my eyes. As a professional photographer, my eyes are the key to my artistry, my biggest asset to my creativity. I found myself dropping back into overthinking mode.

I had well-meaning friends tell me "the surgery is no big deal," even though they had never been through it themselves.

I met with an eye surgeon, and he reviewed the procedure with me. He was surprised to see me in the clinic, as all the other patients in the waiting room were fifteen to twenty years older. He asked if others in my family had cataracts this early. When I said no, he was even more surprised. I asked what causes cataracts. He started listing some of the reasons, and when he hit "long-term use of steroids," I knew the chemo was to blame.

I went through the procedure on the first eye and learned quickly why you need to get the second eye done even if it isn't showing signs of cataracts. For two weeks, it was impossible to read or see anything without covering the eye that wasn't operated on. I had my progressive prescription in one eye and almost perfect vision in the other eye.

I still need to use glasses, $1.50 drug store cheaters when reading close-up, but I made it through surgery in both eyes.

Another remnant of chemo is neuropathy in my feet and slight neuropathy in my fingertips. It makes me clumsy at times. I tend to trip and drop things occasionally. The insides of my shoes always feel like there is something jammed in there, but it's just the strange numbness on the bottom of my feet.

And then there is the scar. My port scar on my upper chest. At first, I wanted to cover it up with a tattoo or something. But then, as I sat with it, I began to like it. It is my battle scar, representing the battle I won.

When I wear lower-cut tops or v-necks, you can clearly see it. I now feel it is a tattoo in its own right, one that shows that I am a survivor. I made it through hell and back. This scar is something I can now embrace.

## Chapter Twenty-Three
# 10 Years Later

I raise monarch butterflies. I grow milkweed in my garden, which attracts a monarch butterfly to come and lay her eggs upon the leaves. Once those eggs hatch and turn into little caterpillars, I collect them and put them into a safe netting to keep predators away. I love this because it allows me to watch their miraculous transformation.

Throughout the caterpillar's life cycle, it goes into stasis and transforms five different times as it sheds its old self and grows into the new, bigger self, stronger than the last version.

Then, when the caterpillar has reached its final stage, it chooses a spot in which to create a chrysalis. The caterpillar goes through its very last transformation, creating a shell in which to transform.

Once the butterfly breaks out of its chrysalis, its wings slowly unfold and expand, as the wings begin to fill with the life force needed for this butterfly to carry on and spread its beauty throughout the garden.

I find this is an incredible metaphor for how we live our lives. We go through many stages, starting in a lack of awareness, then as we grow and we learn more. We then come out stronger and more aware until we reach the place of awakening to our true self, our purpose, our mission here on earth. If we choose, we in essence transform into beautiful butterflies that can spread love and light wherever they go. It may sound cliché, but I feel it is the perfect analogy for how humanity can transform.

There are many things put on this planet in order to create balance. The graceful deer, the cunning fox, the adorable, loving nature of the otter. These are creatures that we all embrace, but for a moment, let's consider the bees, who work and gather for their queen, yet should they be disrupted, they can deliver a nasty sting. Or the snake who is here with a purpose to offer balance in the food cycle. The snake is feared and even deadly at times. Or the vulture who appears to many as a dark and ominous creature, but the vulture assists in cleaning up remains, thus keeping its territory clear of disease.

All creatures, all people, all circumstances, have a place and mission to fulfill on this earth and in this matrix. It doesn't need to be grand; it may be dark and fearful, or it may be simple and uninteresting, but everything here serves a purpose in the intricate architecture of this reality.

So you can do one of two things at this point: you can throw this book in the trash and continue to hold the narrative that you did NOT create this life for yourself, this non-fiction idea of victimhood. Or you can stand up and claim responsibility for your "being" and start feeling and feeding your body, mind, and spirit with beautiful, positive, and joyous thoughts and ideas. These are the stories that a healthy human is made of.

This shift began to happen for me during treatment when I finally saw, really saw with my spirit, all the external toxicity that I had invited into my world. The job that fueled anxiety, resentment, and repressed anger. The marriage that was a constant state of conflict. Two souls who carried so much dense, unresolved trauma that they couldn't even see each other through their cloak of resentment. I carried the unrequited guilt that I raised my children in this cesspool of toxicity, making it challenging for them to ever see what a healthy relationship should be. All these things created my dis-ease. All of these things, plus many more that remain unspoken, contributed to my cancer.

These are not things that I could snap my finger and change overnight, this is a very long road that you have to commit to if you wish to see yourself healthy on the other side. This is not for the faint of heart, you have to summon up the fortitude inside of you. Your soul needs to be screaming at you so loud that you will do whatever it takes to right the wrongs you have created, as you are the creator of your world.

Look at this process as one baby step at a time. And, if you are going to carry your type A personality into this scenario, you will fail. You need to understand you will stumble, you will make many mistakes, but the idea that you are aware of those shortcomings is where you will begin to win this cancer war.

Healing is part of the ongoing human experience. To me, you are only healed to the point to where your vibration is at this moment. On top of that, there should be brain, gut, and heart coherence. All three parts of your human operating system need to be in alignment, holding the unwavering belief that you are joyful, you are healthy, and you are strong.

When I embarked on this writing journey, my body began to sink into physical trauma. I started to have stomach aches, I started to feel nauseous and I started allowing fear of cancer to creep back into my awareness.

Intrinsically, I knew I was strong and healthy. I get out in the woods and I walk 5 to 7 miles almost every day of the week. I have found (and this is strictly personal to me, you would need to do your own investigating of this lifestyle) that being in a state of GKI ketosis, sometimes to dietary or therapeutic levels, has really made me stronger and more "regular" in my daily constitution. This is how I knew my human avatar was operating at the optimal level.

I realized that I needed to tap into my body and examine where feelings were coming from. I am a walking meditator. Sure, I can sit in quiet, but I much prefer to immerse myself deep in nature, disconnect from my brain, and allow the quietness to come in as I am physically moving energy through my body. This is when I receive messages from many glorious, etheric beings that hold pure light and love.

When I tapped into my human body, I found out that I had neglected her, neglected her feelings, and ignored what she was saying to me. I was shocked as well as saddened that I hadn't even thought to tell my body that I was working on a book that encompassed the *past*. She was concerned that the trauma of cancer, the surgery, and the chemotherapy might be starting all over again.

That is when I had to walk away from my writing for several months. I had to take the time to connect with my physical body and work on this part of my healing, the healing that I had neglected to do for the past nine years. I didn't beat myself up over this, I saw it as another incredible piece of awareness being brought to me so I can continue to work on the physical process of my cancer healing.

I spent a good deal of time lying on my back, going through my body in meditation, talking to it, telling it, it was strong and healthy. I told my body how grateful I was for its strength and stamina. I sent her love, so much deep heart-centered love, unconditional love for being the magnificent vessel that she is, and how eloquently she carried me through that year of cancer surgery and chemotherapy. I assured my body that we were in this together now, going forward, bringing forth our highest and best potential for this lifetime.

Through all of my healing work, my research, my consciousness awakening, and my deep self-love that was unfurling, it never occurred to me that I needed to be communicating with my actual physical being. I had neglected her. But no longer!

Every part of us—from the meat suit we were given upon arriving on this planet to our inner self/higher self that is continually tethered to our physical being, and everything in between—all aspects of us that deserve our attention and love. This is what it means to be doing the inner work.

The inner work is you looking inside of you, getting in touch with your physical being and your etheric being, digging deep into the trauma and pain on any and every level of YOU. I am not discounting the external things that come into your life, but looking at those and trying to fix them is not going to get to the root of what your soul is here to accomplish.

I always thought the saying, "Focus on yourself, and everything else around you will fall into place" was trite. It felt too simple, and clearly, I needed a more complex directive (says the recovering type A personality). But after fighting to fix everything in my external world to no avail, I figured I would give it a try.

I dug deep into my inner child. I talked with her, I loved her, I made her feel safe. I dug into the traumas in my field of awareness. I sat with my traumas, I cried over them, I let them move through my entire being, forgave myself, forgave my traumas, and then sent them to the Creator to transmute and deliver them into the light. I studied, I learned, and I listened to my soul. I released my expectations of what I thought my purpose might look like and leaned into the energetic flow of the Universe.

As I started to melt and morph into this different person, situations and people started to fall from my life. This again had me circling back into another newfound trauma of wanting to be liked and needing to belong. Similar situations like this kept rising to the surface over the past ten years. We are always and continually a work in progress. Any spiritual practitioner who proclaims to be more enlightened than you or to know more than you is a false prophet.

I believe we have agreed to come into this lifetime to explore the vast, never-ending aspects of being a human in the third dimension. To learn how to disconnect from the external, move into the internal, and expand our heart and soul into a state of unconditional love. That, my friend, is no simple task.

Another aspect of my healing was learning how to forgive (but not forget) those who dismissed me, rejected me, and kicked me while I was down with cancer. It took me several years to truly embrace forgiveness and even find gratitude for what I received from each of those people in my life. As I tapped into two prominent situations, I saw souls that were wounded and hurting. It was heartbreaking to witness, but it was a portrait that I needed to see in order to move through those final stages, taking my anger and hurt, and moving those feelings into forgiveness, then shifting them into gratitude.

If we look at this world as one giant movie or theatrical production, it's easy to see all of the characters that are a part of your play, each of them moving through the dramatic scenes of your life in order to bring your story (your soul) to a happy ending.

I used to believe that I was a victim, that everything was being done to me by others. Then, after my treatment, I attended a weekend seminar where I shared my story of cancer. The moderator said to me, "You need to stop playing the victim role. Why do you think you're the victim and everything is being done to you?"

That blew my mind wide open. Of course, I was angry at first, believing that the moderator did not see the real me. Clearly, she did not understand that I suffered this incredibly tragic event! That night, when I went home, I couldn't sleep because that victim comment kept running through my mind. That's when my inner self intervened.

I was shown that perhaps my choice in family, my choice in my career, my choice in marriage, and my choice in the people I chose to surround myself with were the root cause of my dis-ease (disease). My attitude, my anger, my victimhood, my trauma and drama, my sadness, my wounded heart, my inability to see the light. All these things *were* the reason I manifested cancer. And in order to move forward, I had to work on and release all those things I listed and more!

I know the line "I manifested my cancer" will trigger a few folks. Follow me down this road of thought for a moment if you would. Imagine yourself as an etheric being out in the void, co-mingling with Source/Creator/God—all joyful and blissed-out, floating in a pool of absolute love all day, every day. Ahhh, sounds quite magnificent to me. However, after a while, you might get a little bored. And now you're watching the beings on this planet and saying to yourself, "Wow, that might be really cool to experience! I wonder what it would be like to _____ " (fill in the blank with the trauma of your choice). Now, I believe when we come here, those things we may want to "experience" are really a contractual obligation for us to fulfill. However, I do believe we all have free will, and if we were able to tap into the awareness of what we signed up for upon arrival to Planet Earth, perhaps we would be able to change that contract through our awareness and through the assistance of our inner self and our spirit guides. But the majority of us come to this planet with absolutely no remembrance of the incredible souls we are. We exchange our eternal knowledge for amnesia in order to feel the full experience of this rollercoaster ride called Planet Earth.

When I connect deeply into my soul, I do believe I came here to experience cancer and everything that went along with everything I have described in this book. If I did not have this journey, my consciousness would not have expanded to the level of awareness that I currently hold.

It is also possible that I signed up for this cancer journey to be a living example to other actors in my movie production, so perhaps it would inspire or enlighten them in some way.

I say this as something for you to consider, not as something that makes me better than anyone else. You see, another one of the big things that we forget when we come here is that we are all one unified field. We are all bound together by a golden thread, we are all ascended masters; otherwise, we would not have come to this planet in this time. Each of us, good or bad, is an important cog in this wheel of life.

Another belief I hold is that everyone on Earth is here to assist in the planet's ascension. To me, this does not mean we are all gonna eventually float out of our bodies and fly up into heaven, we are actually here to create heaven on Earth. We are here to usher out the old patriarchal way of operating and usher in a new, more harmonious existence. Please don't ask me what that would look like because we each have our own ideas around what would create harmony and heaven on Earth. And I like to believe that each of us can have that version of heaven on earth if we choose.

Will I see this in my lifetime? Probably not. However, I have already seen great strides in humanity, and conversely, I have also seen very malevolent and cruel sides of humanity as well. The Ying and Yang. The good and bad. Coexisting as one on this glorious disco ball floating in the universe.

Before I get too far off track, these are just a smattering of the thought processes and ideas that have come up for me during my exploration of self. All this led me to where I am today.

I am not a guru, nor do I ever wish to be. I am simply a girl standing here telling you the intimate details of my cancer journey. This journey will be ongoing for the rest of my life as my soul continues to explore and expand.

Perhaps some of these ideas will resonate for you. Maybe it will open up a rabbit hole for you to explore. Wherever you go or wherever you land after reading this book, I see the highest and best outcome for your journey as you find YOUR Zen with cancer.

God I love this life!
AND I love you!
xoxo Linda

## Chapter Twenty-Four
# Visualize Yourself Cancer-Free

I now invite you to go on a meditative journey with me. No matter where you are in your cancer journey, whether you are the patient, the caregiver for the loved one, you are welcome to join.

Meditation is a wonderful way to calm the thinking mind and tap into your soul self. Guided meditations are great for those who are challenged in calming the mind chatter. Guided meditations are also great to take you on a calming journey and integrate healing energies.

You can read this meditation or listen to an audio version at:

theowlandthecrone.com/cancerclearingmeditation.

Close your eyes, take three deep cleansing breaths, in through the nose and out through the mouth.

Feel your energy drop down from your headspace, clearing all thoughts that you carry in this now moment. Bring that clear and pure energy center that you have created down into your heart space. Breathing through the nose and out through your mouth in long, slow, deep breaths. With every out breath release any negative thought forms and feel your heart expanding, expanding past your body, expanding into the space of your room, expanding out into your neighborhood, keep expanding until you feel you can expand no more.

Now, I want you to invite in all the benevolent beings from the etheric realms that support you on your earthly journey. These may be your guardian angels, they may be spirit guides, they may be loved ones who have crossed to the other side. Do not concern yourself with identifying these beings at this moment you may have an inner knowing, but just set time aside for now. Ask your benevolent team that is with you now to illuminate the path ahead of you. Ask them to clearly pave this path for you with golden iridescent Christed light, look down that path, and observe what you see in front of you.

Are your guides showing you shifts that you inherently know would assist you on this journey? Are you seeing changes that you need to make, now illuminated? Are you hearing that your current path does not serve your highest and best good? Can you smell where the toxicity still resides in your energy body? Take note of everything that you see. Do not judge any of it; simply observe it. Observe it with neutrality. Observe it as if you were witnessing this in a stranger. These neutral observations serve as a guide, leading you toward complete mental, physical, and spiritual healing. Allow the angels and guides to show you where you can make changes for your human body, the container in which your soul resides.

Now invite your guides, angels, and loved ones who have crossed over into your field to assist you and guide you toward the highest and best outcome for your human. Ask them to illuminate the lessons that you are to learn from this experience. Ask them to assist you in gently receiving completion of this lesson and embodying all that it was meant to teach you so that you may now move forward with a strong, healthy mind, body, and spirit.

Sit with this vision. Start at the crown, which is the top of your head, and slowly imagine a beautiful golden iridescent light filling every cell of your body as you move from the crown through your forehead, igniting the connection to God/Source.

Now, moving down into your third eye, on your forehead, between your physical eyes, illuminating all the truths that you carry deep within your soul.

Slowly move down through your mouth and into your throat, igniting in your truth, the truth that you have been afraid to speak. This is an important area that may be blocked if you have been feeling repressed and unable to speak your desires and truth.

Continue with deep, slow breaths and move slowly down into your heart space, which resides in the center of your chest. It emits a beautiful green, emerald aura from your spirit. Sit in your heart space for a moment and just *feel*. What are those feelings that you have pushed to the back of your heart space? Breathe deep and bring them forward now.

Know that you are worthy, you are a God-spark, you are completely loved at the purest, deepest, and most unconditional level. Your soul holds this within. Invite this forward in an act of deep self-love for your humanity. Embody this with each breath, as *you* are a divine and perfect being, just as you are. Breathe. Slow, deep breaths in through the nose and out through the mouth. If you need to release tears, let them flow. Release anything that comes up for you in the now moment.

Once you are ready, you can continue down past the heart space into what is known as the solar plexis area, just below the ribcage to your belly button. This is where our true brain resides. This is where we feel our gut instincts warn us, guide us, and direct us to what is best for our being. This area goes largely ignored any time that you override these instinctual feelings and ignore what needs to happen.

Invite in the beautiful light to your solar plexis, tell your gut-brain that you will promise to listen. Ask your guides to assist you in knowing when your solar plexis is trying to communicate with you.

Now, continue to slowly bring this beautiful golden iridescent Christed light down to the bottom of your tailbone to what is known as the root chakra or sacral space. This is the area that keeps you grounded to

Mother Earth; this is where you can deeply feel your connection to the planet and to nature. This is what keeps you from floating to the stars and tethered here to our planet.

Continue down from the base of your spine to your feet. Feel a golden cord connecting to the ground beneath you. This is where you can see guidance from earthly connections, from spirit animals, and from gut observations that you make throughout your day. Imagine the most beautiful crystalline threads shooting out of your feet and making their way through the earth to Mother Earth/Gaia's core.

Breathe deep in through the nose and out through the mouth. Everything around you in nature is communicating with you; it is up to you and your inner knowing to receive and discern what those messages are. Everything is given to you for your highest and best good unless you are consciously choosing otherwise.

Now slowly come back up through your beautiful, light-filled body, back up through your legs, through your spine, past your gut, into your heart space, through your throat and up to your third eye, and through the crown, you are beautifully connected now to all realms of the highest, purest, iridescent, golden Christed light.

Whether your human self is aware or not, you are a Divine being of love and light. Your soul came here to learn many lessons and to assist others in learning lessons as well. Everything is in perfect order.

Choose the highest path for your being; trust that you will be guided. Do not surround yourself with negative thoughts, toxic energies, or undesirable spirits. These will drag you off course. Should you fall, ask for assistance from your angels and guides; they are here to serve but need to be invited in to do so.

Now, let's take three deep cleansing breaths. When you open your eyes, you are going to feel centered and energized, ready to receive complete healing for your mind, body, and spirit. You will be instinctually guided how to move forward and receive continual healing. You will be given assistance along the way. Feel into that guidance, and only go with what resonates for you and your soul. Breathe deep again, and when you are ready, open your eyes.

If you feel the need to rest after this meditation, honor your body and do so. Sit in quiet, drink lots of water, keep yourself out of your headspace and in your heart space as long as possible as you move forward. This takes time, years, even decades, of practice, so be patient and just keep doing your best.

I love you!
Linda

# Acknowledgments & Gratitude

I am grateful for my cancer journey and all who supported me on my road to healing. Everyone who sent a message, called, mailed a card or care package, or paid a visit will always be held dear to me. Your love, caring, and support lifted me up in my darkest hours. I would not be here if it wasn't for your kindness and compassion.

I couldn't imagine venturing into this cancer journey without my amazing husband, Greg Stansberry, by my side. Having deep, unconditional love from someone when you are cast into the unknown is powerful medicine. We cried, laughed, fought, prayed, walked through fire, and spit on the devil, and here we are, alive and kicking! I am grateful that I have found the one my soul loves. Baby, there is nothing we cannot get through together.

My gratitude is unending for the support of the beautiful babies that I love so dearly. I am one blessed mom. My eldest son, Alex—you are so intelligent, strong, handsome, with a fierce wit. You are an incredibly caring and loyal soul to all those you love. I am proud of all that you have overcome and the conscience and caring man that you have become. I am honored to be called your "Ma."

Hannah, my beautiful, funny, bright, empathetic, and intuitive daughter—I see your Light. You are an amazing beacon that shines luminous in this crazy world. I am so very grateful for you and for you giving us our grandson Robbie, he brings us immense joy. I cannot wait to be MOB at your wedding as you and Rob become Mr. & Mrs. My heart sings for you, baby girl! You deserve ALL the joy!

My baby boy, Noah, no matter how old you get, you will forever be my beautiful baby boy. You make me laugh with your voice impersonations and sense of humor—they are beautiful gifts. I hope you find happiness, peace, and your place in this world. Know that above all else in your life, you have a mother who deeply loves you beyond measure.

I never imagined I would have more children until two beautiful, determined, and intelligent ladies entered my life when I reunited with Greg. I love them fiercely as if they were my own.

Bonus daughter Megan, you are so kind and caring. I appreciate that I have another fearless travel companion, and adventurous foodie who is willing to partake in the decadence of life with me. You are witty beyond your years. I couldn't ask for more, but wait, there's more! You have a massive, elephant-size heart and a wild, Gypsy soul. I am blessed to call you a daughter.

Bonus daughter Melissa, your love, care, and compassion for animals fill my heart with so much joy. You are the most tenacious person I know. Your ability to pivot and succeed every time is amazing to witness.

You are clearly a manifestor for sure. And the icing on the cake is sweet Georgia Lee, our beautiful and bright granddaughter. You and Brandon definitely have your hands full with that lil' ginger girl.

I also wish to thank my amazing publishing team of Sue Urda and Kathy Fyler. I have felt so loved and supported by you and your team through this whole process. And big thanks to my intuitive editor, Dana Micheli, who lovingly supported and held my words in her heart and hands.

And to my tribe, who over the past ten years told me I needed to mold my musings into a book, I am eternally grateful for your consistent encouragement.

My acknowledgments would not be complete without giving a shout-out to Cat Mulder. You entered my life knowing you had a mission. The companionship, love, and healing you have brought me is immeasurable. Even when you are a big Ass-Cat, you keep me on my toes. I love you.

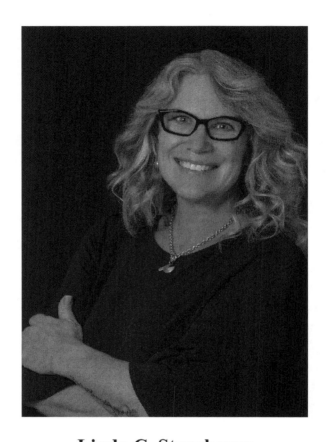

**Linda C. Stansberry**
Photographer. Writer. Artist.
Intuitive. Spiritual Teacher.
Thought Leader.
Podcaster. Blogger.

# About the Author

After leaving her corporate television career, Linda Stansberry fulfilled her dream of becoming a small business owner, running a successful photography studio, LindaStansberryPhotography.com.

Linda is an intuitively connected spiritual practitioner, offering guidance and coaching, as well as working with clients via a variety of metaphysical modalities that can be found on her website TheOwlandtheCrone.com. She recently channeled her first Oracle Card Deck, SoulScripts, designed to assist the user in unlocking and activating their own intuitive abilities.

Her highly acclaimed podcast, Conversation for the Soul, is broadcast on over a dozen podcast platforms, including Apple, Spotify, Amazon, and YouTube. She believes stories make great teachers. Her mission is to show people that unfolding a deeper relationship with their higher self will assist an individual in reaching their soul's potential by living a more intuitive and conscious life.

Writing is also part of Linda's calling. Her most notable blog, Finding Zen with Cancer, serves as the launchpad for this book of the same name.

If you are interested in booking a session, you can connect with Linda directly via her email, TheOwlandTheCrone@gmail.com.

Made in the USA
Columbia, SC
14 October 2023